Dismantle or Defuse?

A Comparative Guide to I-CBT and ACT for
Treating OCD and Obsessional Thinking

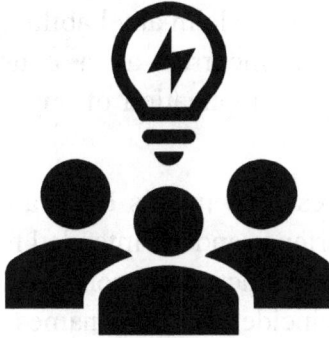

Mable Jacquard McGowan

First Edition

ISBN: 978-1-923604-69-8

This book is intended as an educational guide and theoretical resource for qualified mental health professionals. It is not a substitute for formal clinical training, supervision, or professional judgment. The application of the therapeutic techniques described herein requires appropriate professional qualifications and adherence to the ethical guidelines and legal requirements of the practitioner's jurisdiction.

The information provided does not constitute medical advice and is not intended for self-diagnosis or self-treatment by the general public. The publisher and author disclaim any liability, loss, or risk, personal or otherwise, which is incurred as a consequence, directly or indirectly, of the use and application of any of the contents of this book.

All case examples presented in this book are fictional composites based on clinical experience and are intended for illustrative purposes only. Any resemblance to actual persons, living or dead, or actual events is purely coincidental. All names, characteristics, and identifying details have been significantly altered.

Table of Contents

Preface

For many years, the world of therapy offered a fairly standard set of instructions for dealing with difficult thoughts. The advice was often to challenge them, to correct them, or to face the fears they created head-on. For many people, these approaches were life-changing. But for others, they didn't quite work. The struggle continued, and the feeling of being stuck remained.

But the world of psychology is not static. It is constantly growing, learning, and finding new ways to understand the complexities of the human mind. In recent years, a new wave of therapies has emerged, offering fresh perspectives and powerful new tools for those who feel like they've tried everything. This book is about two of the most promising of these new approaches: Inference-Based Cognitive Behavioral Therapy (I-CBT) and Acceptance and Commitment Therapy (ACT).

At first glance, these two therapies could not be more different. One teaches you to become a detective, to carefully investigate the faulty logic that creates your painful thoughts and to dismantle it with evidence and reason. The other teaches you to become a compassionate observer, to learn how to let your thoughts come and go without getting tangled up in them, and to build a life guided by what truly matters to you. One is about dismantling the thought; the other is about defusing from it.

So, which one is right?

That is the question that inspired this book. My goal is not to convince you that one approach is superior to the other. It is to offer you a clear, honest, and practical guide to both. This book is built on the belief that there is no one-size-fits-all solution to human suffering. The path to freedom is a personal one, and you are the one who is best equipped to choose it.

In the Dismantle or Defuse we will explore the worlds of I-CBT and ACT side-by-side. We will break down their core philosophies, learn their key techniques, and see how they can be applied to the real-life struggles that so many of us face. We will use simple language, relatable examples, and practical exercises to make these powerful ideas accessible and useful.

This book is not a substitute for therapy, but it is a roadmap. It is a guide to help you understand the options that are available, to think critically about what might work for you, and to take the first steps toward a new relationship with your own mind. Whether you find your answers in the logical clarity of I-CBT, the mindful acceptance of ACT, or a blend of both, my hope is that this book will empower you with the knowledge and the tools you need to stop struggling and start living. The journey may be challenging, but new and effective approaches are being forged every day, and a freer, more meaningful life is possible.

Mable Jacquard McGowan

The Evolving Landscape of Cognitive Therapy

You've probably felt this before. A thought pops into your head, uninvited and unwelcome, and it just… sticks. It might be a worry about something you did or didn't do, a fear of something that *could* happen, or a nagging doubt that you just can't shake. Soon, that one thought starts playing on a loop, getting louder and more convincing each time. Before you know it, you're caught in a mental trap, spending all your energy trying to argue with the thought, push it away, or do something—anything—to make the anxiety go away.

This is the experience of being stuck in obsessional thinking. It feels like your own mind has turned against you, and you're left trying to navigate a storm inside your own head. For decades, people have been told there are specific ways to handle this, certain rules to follow. But what if the old rules don't work for you? What if the standard advice just makes you feel more anxious or misunderstood?

The good news is that our understanding of the mind is always growing. The ways we approach difficult thoughts and feelings have changed, offering new hope and new strategies for people who feel like they've tried everything. This book is about exploring that new landscape. It's a guide to two of the most powerful modern approaches for dealing with sticky, obsessive thoughts. They are very different from each other, but both offer a path toward freedom. We're going to look at them side-by-side, so you can understand how they work and discover what might finally work for you.

The Post-CBT World

For a long time, the main tool for dealing with difficult thought patterns was something called *Cognitive Behavioral Therapy*, or CBT. The idea behind CBT is simple but powerful: your thoughts,

3

feelings, and behaviors are all connected. If you have a negative thought (like "I'm going to mess this up"), it leads to a negative feeling (like anxiety), which then leads to a certain behavior (like avoiding the situation altogether). CBT teaches you to catch those negative thoughts and challenge them. It's like becoming a detective for your own mind, looking for the evidence that your negative thoughts aren't 100% true.

CBT was a huge step forward. It gave people practical tools to work with their minds instead of feeling helpless. It showed millions of people that they could change how they felt by changing how they thought and acted.

But as helpful as it was, some people found that it didn't quite get to the root of their problems. For certain kinds of thinking—especially the stubborn, looping thoughts that come with obsession—just challenging the thought wasn't always enough. Sometimes, arguing with a thought just seemed to give it more power.

This led to what some call the "third wave" of therapies. These newer approaches didn't throw out the lessons of CBT, but they added new ideas, like mindfulness, acceptance, and personal values. Instead of focusing only on

changing your thoughts, these therapies started asking a different question: What if you could change your *relationship* to your thoughts? What if you could learn to let them come and go without getting tangled up in them? This shift opened up a whole new world of possibilities for people who felt stuck.

Reflection: Think about a time you tried to argue with a worry. Did it help, or did it feel like you were just adding fuel to the fire? What does this tell you about your own patterns?

Moving Beyond ERP

When it comes to treating Obsessive-Compulsive Disorder (OCD), the most well-known treatment is a specific type of CBT called *Exposure and Response Prevention*, or ERP. The logic of ERP is straightforward: to get over a fear, you have to face it. In ERP, you would gradually expose yourself to the very things that trigger your obsessive thoughts, and then you would actively stop yourself from doing the compulsive ritual you normally do to feel better.

For example, if you have a fear of contamination, you might be asked to touch a doorknob and then not wash your hands for a set amount of time. The idea is that by sitting with the anxiety without "fixing" it, your brain eventually learns that the doorknob isn't actually dangerous and the anxiety will go down on its own. For many people, this approach is incredibly effective and life-changing.

But let's be honest: it can also be terrifying.

Many people hear about ERP and immediately think, "I could never do that." The idea of purposely triggering their worst fears is just too much to handle. As a result, many people either refuse the treatment or drop out before they can see the benefits. For others, ERP helps reduce their compulsions, but they are still left with the nagging, underlying doubt that started the problem in the first place. They may be able to resist washing their hands, but their mind is still screaming at them that they are contaminated.

This is where the need for alternatives becomes so clear. What about the people who aren't ready for ERP? Or the ones who tried it and it didn't work? What if the goal isn't just to tolerate anxiety, but to resolve the doubt that causes the anxiety in the first place? The newer therapies provide answers to these questions. They offer a different way in—one that doesn't always require you to walk directly into the storm of your greatest fear.

Dismantle or Defuse?

This brings us to the heart of this book and the two modern approaches we will explore: *Inference-based Cognitive Behavioral Therapy (I-CBT)* and *Acceptance and Commitment Therapy (ACT)*. They both help with obsessional thinking, but they do it in completely opposite ways. The core difference comes down to one question:

When a painful, obsessive thought shows up, should you **dismantle** it or **defuse** from it?

The I-CBT Approach

I-CBT says that obsessive thoughts aren't just random, intrusive thoughts that you misinterpret. It argues that these thoughts are the end result of a faulty reasoning process. It's a specific mental habit where you start to trust your imagination more than you trust your own senses and reality. You build a whole story in your head—an "obsessional narrative"—that feels completely real, even though there's no actual evidence for it in the here and now.

The goal of I-CBT is to help you become a detective who investigates that faulty reasoning. You don't challenge the *content* of the thought (e.g., "Are my hands really dirty?"). Instead, you challenge the *process* that led to the thought in the first place (e.g., "How did I get from seeing clean hands to being certain they are contaminated?").

You learn to see that the obsessive doubt is based on a fictional story, not on reality. Once you see that the reasoning behind the doubt is flawed, the doubt itself collapses. And when the doubt is gone, the anxiety and the urge to do compulsions simply dissolve because there's no longer a reason for them to be there.

In I-CBT, you **dismantle** the thought by showing that the foundation it was built on is faulty. You prove to yourself that the doubt was never valid to begin with.

The ACT Approach

ACT takes a completely different path. It suggests that trying to fight, change, or dismantle your thoughts is often the very thing that keeps you stuck. The problem isn't that you have negative thoughts— everyone has them. The problem is that you get *fused* with them. You treat them as absolute truths or urgent commands that you must obey.

The goal of ACT is not to change the thought, but to change your relationship with it. You learn to *defuse* from your thoughts, which means seeing them for what they are: just words, images, and sensations passing through your mind. You don't have to believe them or fight them. You can just notice them, acknowledge their presence, and then gently shift your focus back to what you actually care about in your life—your values.

ACT teaches you to accept the presence of uncomfortable thoughts and feelings without letting them run your life. The goal isn't to feel good all the time; it's to live a rich and meaningful life, even when difficult thoughts and feelings show up.

In ACT, you **defuse** from the thought by stepping back and seeing it as just a thought, robbing it of its power to control your actions. You make the thought irrelevant.

Let's look at a quick example. Imagine someone is stuck on the thought, "What if I accidentally leave the stove on and the house burns down?"

- An **I-CBT** approach would help them see the faulty reasoning: "I see the stove is off. My senses tell me it's off. The thought that it *might* be on is coming from an imaginary story, not from reality. That story is not reliable, so I can dismiss the doubt."

- An **ACT** approach would help them unhook from the thought: "There's that 'stove story' again. I notice my mind is generating this thought. I'm not going to argue with it. I'm just going to thank my mind for trying to keep me safe, and then I'm going to focus on what matters to me right now, which is reading a book to my child."

As you can see, both paths can lead to freedom, but they take you on very different journeys.

Who This Book Is For

This book is for you if you feel like you're in a constant battle with your own mind. It's for you if you're tired of being bossed around by worry, doubt, and fear. It's for you if you've tried other things that haven't worked, or if the standard advice just doesn't feel right for you.

You don't need a formal diagnosis to benefit from these ideas. This is for anyone who struggles with:

- Thoughts that get stuck on a loop.

- Constant worrying about "what if" scenarios.

- The need to check things over and over.

- Avoiding situations because of a persistent fear.

- Feeling like you can't trust yourself or your own judgment.

My goal is not to tell you which approach is "better." The truth is, what works for one person might not work for another. Instead, my goal is to give you a clear, honest, and practical guide to both I-CBT and ACT. We will break down each approach into simple, understandable steps. We will use real-life examples and provide exercises you can start using right away.

By the end of this book, you will have a deep understanding of two very different but equally powerful toolkits for your mind. You will be able to make an informed choice about which path feels right for you, or even how you might be able to use ideas from both. This is about empowering you with knowledge and options, so you can finally stop fighting with your mind and start living your life.

With this foundation established, we will first explore the world of I-CBT, learning how to become a detective for our own thoughts and dismantle the stories that keep us stuck.

Chapter 1: Foundational Principles of I-CBT

Most of us have been taught to think about anxiety in a certain way. The story usually goes like this: a strange or scary thought pops into your head, you take it too seriously, and that overreaction is what causes all the problems. For years, the solution was to challenge that thought, to argue with it, or to prove it wrong. But what if that's not the whole story? What if the problem isn't the thought itself, but the faulty mental process that created it in the first place?

This is where a newer approach, *Inference-Based Cognitive Behavioral Therapy (I-CBT)*, comes in. It offers a completely different way of looking at obsessive thinking. Instead of focusing on your reaction to a scary thought, I-CBT goes back to the very beginning and asks, "How did your brain even come up with this doubt?" It suggests that the sticky, looping thoughts that cause so much distress aren't just random mental noise. They are the end product of a specific, flawed reasoning process.

Think of it like being a detective at a crime scene. Traditional therapy might focus on dealing with the aftermath—the mess, the chaos, the emotional fallout. I-CBT, on the other hand, goes looking for the first clue. It wants to figure out the exact moment things went off track. By understanding the faulty logic that started the whole chain reaction, you can solve the mystery at its source. Once you see how the trick works, the illusion loses its power. This chapter is about understanding the foundational ideas of this powerful approach.

A Paradigm Shift

For a long time, the gold standard for therapy, Cognitive Behavioral Therapy (CBT), operated on a simple but effective idea: our thoughts, feelings, and behaviors are all connected. The core theory behind

CBT for obsessive thoughts is that the problem starts with a normal, intrusive thought—the kind everyone has—that you then *misinterpret* or *appraise* as being dangerous or significant .For example, a passing thought like, "What if I didn't lock the door?" is seen as normal. It only becomes a problem when you attach a catastrophic meaning to it, like, "If I didn't lock the door, my family will be in danger, and it will be all my fault." The therapy, then, focuses on challenging that catastrophic appraisal.

I-CBT represents a major shift from this way of thinking. It proposes something radical: **the obsessive thought isn't a normal thought that you misinterpret; it's an abnormal doubt that comes from a faulty reasoning process**. The problem isn't your

appraisal of the thought; the problem is the flawed logic that *created* the thought to begin with.

So, in the case of the locked door, traditional CBT would focus on the belief, "It would be catastrophic if the door were unlocked." I-CBT, however, goes back a step further. It asks, "Why do you doubt the door is locked in the first place, especially when you have a memory of locking it?" It targets the mental leap you made from reality (seeing the locked door) to a fictional possibility ("but what if it's not?"). This is a fundamental difference. I-CBT isn't about managing your reaction to a thought; it's about correcting the faulty reasoning that produces the thought itself. It's a shift from focusing on the

meaning of the thought to focusing on the *mechanics* of how the thought was built.

The "Upstream" Intervention

To understand this difference, it helps to use an analogy of a river. Imagine your obsessive thought is a boat heading for a waterfall of anxiety and compulsive behaviors.

Traditional therapies, like Exposure and Response Prevention (ERP), are *downstream* interventions. They wait for the boat (the obsession) to appear and then teach you how to handle the rough waters. They might have you ride out the anxiety without grabbing for the life raft (the compulsion) until the fear subsides. You learn to tolerate the distress. This is a behavioral approach that targets the compulsions and the anxiety that follows the thought.

I-CBT, on the other hand, is an *upstream* intervention. It doesn't wait for the boat to get into dangerous waters. Instead, it goes upstream to the very source of the river and asks, "Who is launching this boat, and why?" I-CBT targets the reasoning process that creates the initial doubt. The core idea is simple and logical:

if you can prove that the initial doubt is invalid, then there is no reason for the anxiety or the compulsions to exist. The entire downstream sequence—the fear, the urgency, the need to perform a ritual—is cut off at the source.

This is why I-CBT is considered a cognitive intervention, while ERP is a behavioral one. It's not about learning to tolerate anxiety; it's about demonstrating that the anxiety is based on a false premise. By working upstream, you're not just managing the problem; you're preventing it from ever gaining momentum.

Reflection: Think about one of your own looping worries. Can you trace it back to the very first moment of doubt? What was happening right before that doubt appeared? Were you responding to something real in your environment, or to a "what if" in your mind?

Core Concept — Inferential Confusion

So, what is this faulty reasoning process that I-CBT talks about? The central concept is called *inferential confusion*. This might sound complicated, but the idea is actually quite simple. Inferential confusion is a mental glitch where you get tangled up in imagination and possibility, to the point where you start to distrust your own senses and your direct perception of reality.

It's a process where a story you create in your mind feels more real and more trustworthy than what your eyes and ears are telling you in the present moment. This isn't just about having a good imagination; it's about your imagination completely overriding reality.

Inferential confusion has three key ingredients:

1. **A profound distrust of your senses and yourself.** You might see that your hands are clean, but a voice in your head says, "You can't trust what you see. There could be invisible germs." This is a core feature—a fundamental lack of trust in your own ability to perceive the world accurately.

2. **An over-reliance on imagined possibilities.** The world of "what if" and "might be" becomes more important than the world of "what is." A person with OCD might think, "It's *possible* that I hit someone with my car, even though I didn't feel anything and saw nothing in my rearview mirror." That remote possibility is treated as a probable reality.

3. **Using information out of context.** This is one of the sneakiest parts of inferential confusion. Your brain will grab unrelated facts to support the obsessive doubt. For example, you might have read an article about a rare disease. Later, when you have a minor headache, your mind pulls that out-of-context information and concludes, "This headache could be that rare disease I read about!".

Let's look at a simple case. Someone named John has just checked that the stove is off. He can see with his own eyes that all the knobs are in the "off" position.

- **Reality:** The stove is off.

- **Inferential Confusion:** John's mind starts a story. "Yes, it *looks* off, but what if I bumped a knob without realizing it? I remember reading a story once about a house fire that started from a faulty stove. It's *possible* that could happen to me. I can't trust my eyes; the possibility of a fire is too great."

In this moment, John has stopped trusting his senses (what he sees) and has started living in an imagined story built on remote possibilities and out-of-context information. That is inferential confusion in action. Research has shown that this specific reasoning process is a better predictor of OCD symptoms than the general beliefs often targeted in traditional CBT (Aardema et al., 2022).

Why Exposure is Logically Unnecessary

This brings us to one of the most significant differences between I-CBT and other therapies: **I-CBT does not use exposure therapy**. This isn't because it's trying to be a "gentler" or less scary option. Within the logical framework of I-CBT, exposure is simply unnecessary and irrelevant.

Here's why. Exposure and Response Prevention (ERP) is based on learning theory. It assumes that you have a learned fear response to a trigger (like a doorknob). The goal is to expose you to that trigger without letting you do the compulsion (washing your hands) so that your brain can learn through experience that the trigger is not dangerous. The anxiety is expected to decrease over time through a process called habituation. For this to work, you

have to feel high levels of anxiety.

I-CBT operates on a completely different premise. It argues that the trigger doesn't directly cause anxiety. The trigger activates the faulty reasoning process of inferential confusion, which then creates an obsessional doubt.

It is the doubt—the conclusion that something might be wrong— that is the true source of the anxiety.

Therefore, the therapeutic target in I-CBT is to resolve that initial doubt. If you can successfully learn to see the reasoning as flawed and dismiss the doubt as an irrelevant product of your imagination, the logical basis for the anxiety disappears. There is no longer a valid reason to be anxious.

Think back to John and the stove.

- In an **ERP** model, he would be asked to leave the house without checking the stove again and to sit with the intense anxiety until it fades.

- In an **I-CBT** model, the work is done before he even feels the urge to check. He would learn to recognize the moment his mind jumps from the reality of the off-stove to the imaginary story of a fire. He would learn to say to himself, "That's an obsessional doubt. It's not based on my senses; it's based on a fictional story. I can trust what I see."

Once he does that, the doubt is resolved. And if there's no doubt, there's no anxiety to habituate to. Forcing him to do an exposure would be pointless because the goal isn't to learn to tolerate the fear of a fire; it's to show him that, based on the evidence of reality, there is no valid reason to fear a fire in the first place. This makes I-CBT a powerful alternative for the many people who find the high levels of distress required for ERP to be a barrier to treatment (Wolf et al., 2024).

A Different Path Forward

- I-CBT proposes that obsessive thoughts are not normal thoughts you misinterpret, but abnormal doubts created by a faulty reasoning process. The focus is on fixing the *process*, not just challenging the *thought*.

- It works "upstream" by targeting the source of the doubt. If the initial doubt can be resolved, the anxiety and compulsions that follow have no logical reason to exist.

- The core problem is *inferential confusion*, a mental habit where you trust imagination and possibility more than your own senses and the reality in front of you.

14

- Because I-CBT aims to resolve the doubt that causes the anxiety, it does not require exposure therapy. The goal is to show that the anxiety is based on a false premise, not to learn how to tolerate it.

Now that we understand the core theory—that a faulty reasoning process is the engine behind obsessive thinking—we can begin to look at how this plays out in real life. The next step is to learn how to identify the specific parts of this process, including the fictional stories we tell ourselves and the roles we imagine we might play in them.

Chapter 2: The I-CBT Formulation in Practice

Understanding the theory behind I-CBT is one thing, but seeing how it works in practice is where things really start to click. It's like learning the rules of a game versus actually playing it. I-CBT isn't just an interesting idea; it's a practical, step-by-step method for taking apart the machine of obsessive thinking. It gives you a framework to understand your own unique patterns, almost like creating a personal map of your mind.

This process is about more than just identifying a "thinking error." It's about uncovering the entire story that your mind has built to make a doubt feel real and urgent. This story has characters, a plot, and a whole lot of convincing (but faulty) evidence. In this chapter, we're going to learn how to become experts on our own obsessive thoughts. We'll look at the three key components of the I-CBT formulation: deconstructing the story that fuels the doubt, identifying the scary character you're afraid of becoming, and reconnecting with the real, capable person you already are. By the end, you'll see how these pieces fit together to keep you stuck—and, more importantly, how you can start to pull them apart.

Deconstructing the Obsessional Narrative

At the heart of every obsessive doubt is a story. It's not just a random thought; it's a full-blown *obsessional narrative*. This is a compelling, internally consistent, and highly detailed story that your mind creates to convince you that a doubt is real and that you should not trust your senses. The first step in I-CBT is to learn how to see this story for what it is: a piece of fiction.

You and your therapist (or you, with this workbook) become detectives, working together to map out this narrative. You're not

16

trying to argue with the story or prove it wrong. At this stage, you're just trying to understand it. You want to see exactly how it's constructed, what pieces of "evidence" it uses, and what logical tricks it employs to seem so believable.

An obsessional narrative usually pulls from several sources to build its case:

- **Real but irrelevant facts:** It might take a true fact, like "some illnesses start with mild symptoms," and apply it out of context to your current situation.

- **Hearsay or things you've read:** It might use a news story you saw about a freak accident to make that accident seem like a personal, immediate threat.

- **Past experiences:** It might bring up a time you made a mistake in the past as "proof" that you are likely to make a catastrophic mistake now.

- **An over-reliance on possibility:** The story is filled with words like "might," "could," and "what if," treating the most remote possibilities as if they are certainties.

By laying out all the pieces of the story, you start to see it from a distance. You're no longer trapped inside the narrative; you're looking at it from the outside. This process of deconstruction robs the story of its power because you begin to see that it's just a collection of thoughts stitched together in a particular way—not a reflection of reality.

Action Point: Start Mapping Your Story

1. Pick one of your recurring obsessive doubts.

2. On a piece of paper, write down the main "headline" of the story (e.g., "The story that I am contaminated and will make my family sick").

3. Now, list all the "evidence" your mind uses to support this story. Don't judge it; just write it down. Does it use things you've read? Memories? "What if" scenarios?

4. Look at your list. How much of this "evidence" is based on what you can see, hear, and touch in the present moment? How much of it is based on imagination, memory, or possibility?

Identifying the "Feared Self"

Every good story needs a main character, and the obsessional narrative is no exception. In I-CBT, this character is called the *feared self*. The feared self is the nightmarish version of who you are afraid of becoming if the obsession were true. It's the identity that the obsessive story is trying to pin on you.

The feared self is not who you actually are. It's a caricature, a distorted and terrifying version of you that exists only within the obsessional narrative. Here are some common examples of the feared self:

- **The Irresponsible Person:** The one who leaves the stove on, forgets to lock the door, or makes a careless mistake that harms others.

- **The Contaminated Person:** The one who is dirty, spreads germs, and makes loved ones sick.

- **The Dangerous Person:** The one who might lose control and harm someone, either accidentally or on purpose.

- **The Immoral Person:** The one who has secret, unacceptable thoughts and is therefore a bad person.

- **The Vulnerable Person:** The one who is weak, can't cope with illness, and will fall apart at the first sign of trouble.

This feared self is incredibly active within the obsessional story. It's the voice that whispers, "If you don't check that lock one more time, you will be the irresponsible person whose house gets robbed." The story uses the feared self to create a sense of urgent, personal threat.

The problem isn't just that something bad might happen; it's about what it would mean about *you* if it did.

The goal here is to learn to recognize the feared self when it shows up. By giving it a name and understanding its role in the story, you can start to separate it from your true identity. You can learn to see it as a fictional character that OCD created, not as a reflection of who you really are.

Strengthening the "Real Self"

If the feared self is the villain of the story, then the hero is the *real self*. The real self is who you are outside of the obsessional narrative. It's the you that is grounded in your actual life experiences, your values, your common sense, and your senses. While the feared self is built on a foundation of imagination and fear, the real self is built on a foundation of reality.

When you're caught in an obsessive loop, the voice of the feared self can get so loud that it drowns out the voice of your real self. You forget that you are a generally responsible person who has successfully locked the door thousands of times. You forget that you are a caring person who would never intentionally harm anyone. The obsessional narrative makes you lose touch with your own common sense and your own history.

A huge part of I-CBT is actively working to strengthen your connection to your real self. This provides a powerful anchor that can keep you grounded when the storm of the obsessional narrative hits. It's about rebuilding trust in yourself—your senses, your judgment, and your character.

Techniques for strengthening the real self often involve:

- **Clarifying your core values:** What is truly important to you in life, outside of OCD? (e.g., kindness, creativity, family, learning).

- **Recalling evidence from your past:** Making a list of all the times you have acted in line with your real self (e.g., times you were responsible, caring, or competent).

- **Practicing self-compassion:** Learning to talk to yourself with the same kindness you would offer a friend, especially when you're struggling.

The stronger your connection to your real self becomes, the less believable the feared self will seem. You'll have a solid, reality-based identity to stand on, which makes it much easier to see the obsessional narrative as the fiction it is.

Case Study: Sarah's Story of Contamination

Let's put all these pieces together with a detailed example. Sarah is a new mother who has developed an intense fear of contamination. She is constantly worried that she will bring germs into the house and make her baby sick.

1. Deconstructing Her Obsessional Narrative:

Sarah's main obsessional doubt is, "What if my hands are contaminated, and I make the baby ill?" When we map out her narrative, we find it's built on several pieces of "evidence":

- She once read an article about how fragile a newborn's immune system is (a real but out-of-context fact).

- She saw a news report about a flu outbreak in another city (hearsay).

- She remembers getting a bad stomach flu once after eating at a restaurant (a past experience).

- Her story is full of possibilities: "The grocery cart *might* have had germs on it. I *could* have touched something contaminated without realizing it. What if I didn't wash my hands well enough?"

Notice that none of this is based on the present moment. When she looks at her hands, they look clean. But her narrative tells her not to trust her eyes.

2. Identifying Her Feared Self:

Sarah's feared self is "The Negligent Mother." This is the character in her story who doesn't take proper precautions, who carelessly exposes her fragile baby to danger, and who would be solely to blame if the baby got sick. This feared self is what makes the doubt so painful and urgent. It's not just about germs; it's about her identity as a mother. The narrative whispers, "If you don't wash your hands again, you are a bad, negligent mother."

3. Strengthening Her Real Self:

To counter this, Sarah works on reconnecting with her real self.

- **Her Values:** She identifies her core values as being loving, protective, and responsible.

- **Her Reality:** She makes a list of all the things she does every day that prove she is a loving, protective, and responsible mother. She feeds the baby, changes diapers, cuddles him, keeps him warm, and has taken him for all his check-ups. This is the *real* evidence of who she is as a mother.

- **Her Common Sense:** She reminds herself that humans have been raising healthy babies for thousands of years in environments far less sterile than her home.

As Sarah gets better at identifying her obsessional narrative and recognizing the character of "The Negligent Mother," she can start to see the doubt for what it is. She can say, "Ah, there's that story again. The one where I'm the Negligent Mother. But that's not who I am. My real self is a careful and loving mother. I can trust what my senses are telling me right now: my hands are clean." By doing this, she is not arguing about the existence of germs. She is dismantling the entire fictional story that created the doubt in the first place.

21

Your Personal Blueprint

- Every obsessive doubt is supported by an *obsessional narrative*—a fictional story your mind creates using out-of-context facts, possibilities, and past experiences. The first step is to map out this story.

- The main character in this story is the *feared self*—the nightmarish version of who you are afraid of becoming. Identifying this character helps you separate it from your true identity.

- The antidote to the feared self is the *real self*, which is grounded in your values, your common sense, and your actual life experiences. Strengthening your connection to your real self builds a powerful anchor in reality.

- By putting these pieces together, you can create a personal formulation or blueprint of how your obsessive thinking works, which is the key to taking it apart.

With these pieces in place, you now have a map of the problem. You can see the story, you can name the characters, and you have a solid foundation in reality to stand on. This understanding is the essential first step. Now, we can move on to the specific, practical tools you can use in the moment to challenge the faulty reasoning process and stay grounded in the real world.

Chapter 3: The I-CBT Toolkit

A Clinician's Guide to Core Techniques

Now that we've mapped the territory of obsessive thinking—understanding the narrative, the feared self, and the real self—it's time to get practical. This is the part where we move from understanding the problem to actively doing something about it. I-CBT is not just a theory; it's a set of skills. Think of this chapter as your toolkit. These are the specific techniques you can use to dismantle inferential confusion in the moment, rebuild trust in your own mind and senses, and learn to tell the difference between a legitimate concern and a fictional doubt.

These tools are designed to be used systematically. They build on each other, creating a powerful new way of relating to your thoughts and to the world around you. We'll start with exercises to ground you in the present moment, then we'll discuss a critical skill for sorting your thoughts, and finally, we'll look at how these techniques fit into the structured I-CBT program. It's important to remember that, like any new skill, these techniques take practice. Be patient with yourself as you learn. The goal is not perfection; it's progress.

Reality-Sensing Exercises

The engine of inferential confusion is a deep distrust of your senses. The obsessional narrative constantly tells you, "You can't trust what you see, hear, or feel. You have to trust this imaginary story instead." The most direct way to fight this is to actively practice trusting your senses again.

Reality-sensing exercises are designed to pull you out of the world of imagination and anchor you firmly in the physical reality of the here and now.

These are not just relaxation techniques; they are data-gathering exercises. You are using them to collect real, sensory evidence that can be used to challenge the fictional story in your head.

Here are two of the most common and effective reality-sensing techniques:

1. The 5-4-3-2-1 Grounding Exercise

This is a simple but powerful exercise that forces your brain to pay attention to the present moment by engaging all five of your senses. It's hard to get lost in an imaginary story when you are actively focused on the physical world. You can do this anywhere, anytime you feel the pull of an obsessional doubt.

Here's how it works :

- **Pause** and take a slow breath.

- **Notice 5 things you can SEE.** Look around you and name five things in your environment. Don't just glance; really look. Notice the color of the pen on your desk, the way the light hits the window, the texture of the wall.

- **Notice 4 things you can FEEL.** Bring your attention to the physical sensations in your body. Feel the texture of your chair against your back, the fabric of your sleeves on your arms, the solid ground beneath your feet, the temperature of the air on your skin.

- **Notice 3 things you can HEAR.** Listen carefully to the sounds around you. It could be the hum of a computer, the sound of traffic outside, or even the sound of your own breathing.

- **Notice 2 things you can SMELL.** What can you smell in your environment? Maybe it's the faint scent of coffee or the soap on your hands. If you can't smell anything, just notice the neutral smell of the air.

- **Notice 1 thing you can TASTE.** Bring your awareness to your mouth. Can you taste the lingering flavor of toothpaste or your last drink?

This exercise works because it interrupts the obsessive narrative and reconnects you with your immediate, sensory reality. It reminds your brain that there is a real, tangible world outside of the scary story it's telling.

2. The Present-Moment Check

This technique is a more targeted way to gather evidence against a specific doubt. When you feel an obsessional doubt creeping in, you pause and deliberately ask yourself three questions :

1. **What do I actually know based on my senses right now?** (e.g., "I can see the door is closed. I can feel the keys in my pocket.")

2. **What is my imagination adding to this story?** (e.g., "My imagination is adding the idea that a skilled burglar could have picked the lock without me knowing, or that I only *dreamed* I locked it.")

3. **What is the most simple, reality-based conclusion?** (e.g., "The door is locked. The story about the burglar is just a story.")

This check helps you build confidence in your ability to distinguish thoughts from facts. It trains you to rely on direct evidence rather than getting swept away by fictional scenarios.

Clinical Pitfalls

Now, here's a very important warning. Because obsessive thinking often involves a desperate search for certainty, there is a risk that these reality-sensing exercises can be turned into new compulsions or checking rituals. This is the most common mistake people make when trying these techniques on their own. In fact, one study noted that this happens frequently when people practice without guidance

Here's how to avoid this trap:

- **Use the tool once per doubt.** The purpose of these exercises is to gather data, not to get a feeling of 100% certainty. Use the 5-4-3-2-1 exercise or the Present-Moment Check one time to ground yourself and collect the facts. Then, move on.

- **Do not repeat the exercise.** If you find yourself doing the exercise over and over for the same doubt, you have turned it into a compulsion. Repeating it actually reinforces the idea that your senses can't be trusted the first time, which is the exact opposite of what we're trying to achieve.

- **Aim for reasonable confidence, not absolute certainty.** I-CBT helps you find certainty in the here and now, but it acknowledges that absolute certainty about the future is impossible. The goal is to trust the reasonable evidence your senses provide, not to eliminate every last shred of possibility.

Reflection: Have you ever used a coping skill (like deep breathing or positive self-talk) as a way to try to "get rid of" anxiety? Can you see how that could become a subtle compulsion? How can you approach these new reality-sensing tools as data-gathering exercises instead of anxiety-reducers?

Differentiating Doubts

A central skill in I-CBT is learning to tell the difference between two very different kinds of doubt: *normal doubts* and *obsessional doubts*. This is a game-changer, because once you can accurately categorize a doubt, you know exactly how to respond to it.

Normal Doubts:

- **Are based on real-world evidence or a lack of information.** You might have a normal doubt about whether you locked the door if you were genuinely distracted while leaving the house and truly cannot remember performing the action.

- **Are resolved by checking reality.** The doubt goes away once you go back and check the door and see that it's locked.

- **Are useful.** Normal doubt is a helpful mental function that keeps us safe and helps us solve problems.

Obsessional Doubts:

- **Are based on imagination, not reality.** They always lack any objective, sensory basis in the present moment. An obsessional doubt about the door happens even when you

do remember locking it.

- **Are not resolved by checking reality.** Checking the door might provide a moment of relief, but the doubt comes right back because it was never based on the door in the first place. It was based on the fictional story in your head.

- **Are useless and distressing.** They don't solve any real problems; they just create a loop of anxiety and compulsions.

Learning to apply this distinction is a skill that you build over time. You can start by creating a simple log. When a doubt pops into your head, write it down and then ask yourself: "Is there any evidence from my senses *right now* to support this doubt? Or is it coming from my obsessional narrative?" By practicing this, you train your brain to recognize obsessional doubts as mental junk mail—irrelevant noise that can be safely ignored.

Using the I-CBT Modules

I-CBT is not a random collection of techniques; it's a structured, systematic program. It is typically delivered in a series of about 12 distinct modules, with a full course of therapy lasting anywhere from 18 to 24 sessions (IOCDF, n.d.). Each module builds on the last, guiding you through the process of understanding and dismantling your obsessional reasoning.

While working with a trained I-CBT therapist is the best way to go through the program, it's helpful to know what the general path looks like. The modules guide you through all the concepts we've discussed:

- Early modules focus on psychoeducation, helping you understand the I-CBT model and mapping out your personal obsessional narrative.

- Middle modules teach you the core skills, like reality-sensing and differentiating doubts, and help you identify your feared self and strengthen your real self.

- Later modules focus on applying these skills to more challenging situations and developing a plan to prevent relapse.

There are also official client workbooks and exercise sheets that go along with the modules, which can be incredibly helpful for putting these ideas into practice. Knowing that there is a structured path can be very reassuring. It's not an endless, confusing journey; it's a step-by-step process with a clear beginning, middle, and end.

Your Toolkit for Reality

- *Reality-sensing exercises*, like the 5-4-3-2-1 technique and the Present-Moment Check, are practical tools to pull you out of your imagination and ground you in the physical world.

- It is crucial to use these tools to gather data, not to seek certainty. Avoid the pitfall of turning them into new checking rituals by using them once per doubt and then moving on.

- A key skill is learning to differentiate between *normal doubts* (which are based on reality and are useful) and *obsessional doubts* (which are based on imagination and can be dismissed).

- These techniques are part of a structured, module-based program that guides you step-by-step through the process of recovery.

We have now thoroughly examined the world of I-CBT—a world focused on logic, reality, and dismantling the faulty reasoning that creates doubt. But this is only one of the modern approaches to obsessional thinking. Next, we will turn our attention to a completely different philosophy, one that asks us not to dismantle our thoughts, but to change our relationship to them entirely.

Chapter 4: Foundational Principles of ACT

We spend so much of our lives trying to control things. We organize our homes, plan our days, and work hard to make sure things go the way we want. It's a natural human instinct. So, it only makes sense that we try to apply that same logic to our inner world. When a painful thought or a difficult feeling shows up, our first reaction is usually to try to control it. We try to push the thought away, argue with it, or distract ourselves until the feeling goes away. We treat our own minds like a problem to be solved.

But what if that's the wrong approach? What if the very act of trying to control our thoughts and feelings is what's keeping us stuck? This is the starting point for a powerful and very different approach called *Acceptance and Commitment Therapy*, or ACT.

ACT turns the old advice on its head. Instead of teaching you how to change or get rid of your difficult thoughts, it teaches you how to change your *relationship* with them. It suggests that pain and discomfort are normal, unavoidable parts of a full life, and that true freedom comes not from eliminating them, but from learning to live well alongside them. It's a therapy that isn't about feeling good all the time; it's about building a life that is meaningful to you, even when you don't feel good. In this chapter, we'll explore the foundational ideas of ACT and discover a new way to think about our inner struggles.

The Goal of Psychological Flexibility

The ultimate goal of ACT is not to reduce your symptoms or eliminate your anxiety. The goal is to increase your *psychological flexibility*. This is a fancy term for a very simple and powerful idea.

Psychological flexibility is the ability to stay in contact with the present moment, as it is, and to keep moving toward what's important to you, no matter what difficult thoughts, feelings, or sensations show up.

Think of it like being a tree in a storm. A tree that is too rigid will snap and break in a strong wind. But a tree that is flexible can bend and sway with the wind, and when the storm passes, it is still standing, rooted in the ground. Psychological flexibility is that ability to bend without breaking. It's about being open to your experiences, aware of what's happening right now, and committed to living a life that reflects your deepest values.

This is a radical departure from many other therapies. The goal isn't to win the war with your thoughts; it's to get out of the war altogether. Instead of spending all your energy fighting your inner experience, ACT helps you redirect that energy toward building a life you care about. It's a shift from a life focused on avoiding pain to a life focused on pursuing purpose.

Core Concept — Cognitive Fusion and Experiential Avoidance

According to ACT, much of our psychological suffering comes from two intertwined mental habits: *cognitive fusion* and *experiential avoidance*. Understanding these two concepts is the key to understanding the entire ACT approach.

Cognitive Fusion: Getting Hooked by Your Thoughts

Cognitive fusion is the state of being entangled with or "hooked" by your thoughts. It's when you treat your thoughts as if they are absolute truths or direct commands that you must obey. When you are fused with a thought, you don't experience it as just a thought—a string of words and images in your head. You experience it as reality itself.

Here's an example of fusion:

- **A thought appears:** "I'm a failure."

- **When you're fused with it, you react as if you *are* a failure.** You feel shame, you might avoid trying new things, and you see the world through the lens of that thought. The thought isn't just a thought; it's a fact that defines you.

Our minds are constantly producing thoughts—it's what they do. We have thousands of them every day. Some are helpful, some are neutral, and many are just random nonsense. The problem, from an ACT perspective, isn't that we have negative or painful thoughts. The problem is that we get fused with them. We let them boss us around and dictate how we live our lives. ACT teaches you how to *defuse* from your thoughts—to see them as just thoughts, allowing them to come and go without getting tangled up in them.

Experiential Avoidance: The Struggle with Discomfort

Experiential avoidance is the attempt to avoid, suppress, or get rid of unwanted private experiences, like thoughts, feelings, memories, and physical sensations. It's the natural human tendency to run away from discomfort.

This can look like:

- Avoiding social situations because you're afraid of feeling anxious.

- Drinking alcohol to numb feelings of sadness.

- Constantly checking things to get rid of the feeling of doubt.

- Endlessly distracting yourself with your phone so you don't have to think about a problem.

The paradox is that the more we try to avoid our discomfort, the more it tends to control our lives. Our world gets smaller and smaller as we try to build a life where we never have to feel anything unpleasant. Experiential avoidance is like being stuck in quicksand: our instinct is to struggle and fight to get out, but that struggle is precisely what pulls us in deeper. ACT teaches that the way out is to stop struggling and learn to make room for the discomfort.

Reflection: What are some of the ways you try to avoid uncomfortable feelings? Do you distract yourself, numb out, or avoid certain situations? What has been the long-term cost of this avoidance in your life?

The Role of Values

If you're going to stop struggling with your thoughts and make room for discomfort, you need a very good reason to do so. In ACT, that reason is your *values*.

Values are not the same as goals. Goals are specific outcomes you can achieve and check off a list (like getting a degree or running a marathon). **Values are your chosen life directions.** They are the ongoing qualities of action that you want to bring to your life. They are like a compass that points you in the direction of a meaningful life. You can never "achieve" a value, just like you can never "achieve" north. You can only keep moving in that direction.

Examples of values include:

- Being a loving and present partner.

- Being a creative and expressive person.

- Being a compassionate and supportive friend.

- Being a person who takes care of their health.

- Being a person who is curious and always learning.

In ACT, you are encouraged to get very clear on what truly matters to you, deep in your heart. Your values become the "why" that makes the "how" of dealing with discomfort possible. When you know what you want your life to be about, you are more willing to experience some anxiety or sadness along the way if it means you are moving in a direction that is important to you. For example, if you value connection, you might be willing to feel some social anxiety in order to go to a party and meet new people. Your values give you a reason to be brave.

Acceptance, Not Resignation

One of the biggest misconceptions about ACT is that because it talks about "acceptance," it must be a passive or defeatist therapy. People sometimes hear the word and think it means giving up, resigning yourself to your fate, or just letting your problems walk all over you. This couldn't be further from the truth.

In ACT, *acceptance* does not mean liking or wanting your pain. It means **willingly making room for your uncomfortable thoughts and feelings, without trying to change them or push them away, in the service of living a life you value**.

It's an active, courageous, and often difficult choice. It's the choice to stop fighting the unwinnable war against your own mind and to let your inner experiences be what they are. Acceptance is about dropping the rope in the tug-of-war with your anxiety. When you stop pulling, the struggle ends, and you free up all that energy to do something more useful.

So, acceptance is not resignation. It's the opposite. It's a deeply action-oriented stance. It's about accepting the things you can't control (like the thoughts that pop into your head or the feelings that arise in your body) so that you can put your energy into the things you

can control: your actions. It's about saying, "Okay, anxiety, you can come along for the ride, but you're not driving the car. I am, and I'm driving in the direction of my values."

A New Kind of Freedom

- The goal of ACT is not to eliminate pain but to build *psychological flexibility*—the ability to live a rich, full life even when pain is present.

- Much of our suffering comes from *cognitive fusion* (getting hooked by our thoughts) and *experiential avoidance* (trying to run away from discomfort).

- Your *values* are your chosen life directions. They act as a compass, giving you a reason to move forward even when it's hard.

- *Acceptance* in ACT is not passive resignation. It is an active and courageous choice to make room for discomfort so you can focus on what truly matters to you.

We can now see how these foundational ideas are put into practice. The next chapter will introduce the practical framework that ACT uses to build psychological flexibility. We will explore the six core processes that make up the heart of this therapy and see how they apply to the real-life struggles of the people we're trying to help.

Chapter 5: The ACT Formulation in Practice

Knowing the basic principles of ACT is like knowing the ingredients for a recipe. It's a good start, but you still need to know how to put them all together to make a meal. This chapter is about the recipe. It's where we move from the "what" and "why" of ACT to the "how." We'll look at the practical model that therapists use to help people build psychological flexibility and see how it applies to the kinds of problems that keep people stuck.

We'll start by exploring a technique that often comes at the beginning of therapy—one designed to help people see that their old ways of coping aren't working. Then, we'll introduce the central framework of ACT, a model with six core components that all work together. Finally, we'll revisit our case study of Sarah, the new mother with contamination fears, and see how her struggles look completely different when viewed through the lens of ACT. This will give us a clear, side-by-side comparison with the I-CBT approach we explored earlier.

Creative Hopelessness

This might sound like a strange idea, but one of the first steps in ACT is often to guide someone toward a state of *creative hopelessness*. This doesn't mean making them feel that their life is hopeless. It means helping them see that **their *strategies* for dealing with their pain are hopeless**.

Most people who come to therapy have been trying very hard to solve their problems. They've been fighting their thoughts, avoiding their feelings, and struggling to control their anxiety for years. They've tried everything they can think of—distraction, reassurance, reasoning, willpower—and none of it has worked in the long run. In fact, their efforts to control their inner world have often made things worse, shrinking their lives and exhausting them.

Creative hopelessness is the moment of realization when you see that your control agenda is the problem, not the solution. It's the point where you can finally say, "Okay, everything I've been doing to get rid of this pain hasn't worked. Maybe it's time to try something completely different." It's "creative" because this moment of giving up on the old, unworkable strategies is what opens the door to creativity and a new, more flexible way of living. It's the moment you stop digging the hole you're in and become willing to look for a ladder.

Introducing the Hexaflex

The practical application of ACT is organized around a model called the *Hexaflex*, which outlines the six core processes that work together to create psychological flexibility. These are not steps to be completed in order, but rather a set of interconnected skills that you develop over time.

Think of them as six different muscles. The stronger each one gets, the more psychologically flexible you become.

Here are the six core processes of the ACT Hexaflex:

1. **Acceptance:** This is the skill of willingly making room for uncomfortable thoughts, feelings, and sensations. It's about opening up to your experience instead of fighting it. It's the choice to let your feelings be what they are, without trying to change them.

2. **Cognitive Defusion:** This is the process of separating from your thoughts and seeing them as just thoughts—bits of language and images—rather than as objective truths or commands. It's about unhooking from your thoughts so they have less power over you.

3. **Being Present (or Contact with the Present Moment):** This is the skill of bringing your full attention to the here and now, with an attitude of openness and curiosity. It's about getting out of your head and into your life as it is happening, moment by moment.

4. **Self-as-Context (or The Observing Self):** This is the process of connecting with the part of you that is pure awareness—the part that notices your thoughts, feelings, and experiences but is not defined by them. It's the understanding that you are the sky, not the weather that passes through it.

5. **Values:** This is the process of clarifying what is most important to you, what you want your life to stand for. Your values provide the motivation and direction for your actions.

6. **Committed Action:** This is the skill of setting goals that are guided by your values and taking effective action to achieve them, even when it's difficult. It's about behaving like the person you want to be, one step at a time.

These six processes all support each other. For example, being present helps you notice when you're fused with a thought. Defusion makes it easier to accept a difficult feeling. Acceptance frees you up to take committed action in the direction of your values. Together, they form a comprehensive system for building a more flexible and meaningful life.

Reflection: Look at the six processes of the Hexaflex. Which of these "muscles" feels the weakest for you right now? Which one feels the strongest? What might it be like to strengthen just one of them a little bit?

Case Study: Sarah's Story Through an ACT Lens

In Chapter 2, we looked at the story of Sarah, the new mother with an intense fear of contamination, from an I-CBT perspective. We saw how her problem was framed as a faulty reasoning process (inferential confusion) that was driven by an obsessional narrative and a feared self ("The Negligent Mother").

Now, let's look at Sarah's exact same situation, but this time through the lens of ACT. The formulation of the problem will be completely different.

The ACT Formulation of Sarah's Problem:

From an ACT perspective, Sarah's problem is not that she has faulty reasoning. The problem is that she is stuck in a cycle of cognitive fusion and experiential avoidance that is pulling her away from the life she wants to live.

1. Cognitive Fusion:

Sarah is deeply fused with her thoughts about contamination.

- When the thought "My hands might have germs on them" appears, she doesn't see it as just a thought. She treats it as a literal, urgent threat.

- She is also fused with a set of rules and beliefs about what it means to be a "good mother." Her mind tells her, "A good mother never puts her baby at risk. If you don't wash your hands again, you are a bad mother." She is completely entangled in these thoughts, believing them to be absolute truths.

2. Experiential Avoidance:

Sarah's primary goal is to avoid the feeling of anxiety and doubt. All of her compulsive behaviors are in the service of this avoidance.

- She washes her hands repeatedly not to get them clean (they are already clean), but to get rid of the *feeling* of anxiety.

- She avoids touching certain things (like doorknobs or money) to prevent the *feeling* of contamination from showing up in the first place.

- She asks her husband for reassurance to get a temporary hit of relief from the *feeling* of uncertainty.

Her entire life is becoming organized around this desperate attempt to not feel anxious. This is experiential avoidance in its classic form.

3. Disconnection from Values:

The tragic result of this cycle is that it is pulling Sarah away from what she values most.

- **Her stated value:** To be a loving, present, and connected mother.

- **Her actual behavior:** She is spending hours each day washing her hands, lost in her own head, and feeling disconnected from her baby. She is sometimes so afraid of contaminating him that she hesitates to pick him up and cuddle him. The very actions she is taking to be a "good mother" are preventing her from being the kind of mother she truly wants to be.

The ACT Path for Sarah:

A therapist using ACT would not try to convince Sarah that her hands are clean or that her reasoning is flawed. Instead, the therapy would focus on helping her build psychological flexibility using the six core processes.

- **Acceptance:** She would learn to allow the feeling of anxiety to be present in her body without fighting it.

- **Defusion:** She would practice techniques to unhook from the thought "I might be contaminated," seeing it as just a story her mind is telling her, not a command she has to obey.

- **Being Present:** She would practice bringing her full attention to the present moment with her baby—the sight of his face, the feeling of his skin, the sound of his breathing—instead of being lost in her worries about the future.

- **Self-as-Context:** She would learn to connect with the part of her that is the observer of her thoughts and feelings, recognizing that she is not her anxiety.

- **Values:** She would spend time getting crystal clear on what it means to her to be a loving and present mother.

- **Committed Action:** She would start taking small, deliberate steps in line with her values, such as choosing to read a book to her baby for five minutes, even while the feeling of anxiety is still there.

The goal is not to make the anxiety go away. The goal is to help Sarah live a rich, meaningful life as a mother, and to learn that she can do so even when her mind is generating scary thoughts and her body is feeling anxious.

A Blueprint for Flexibility

- The ACT journey often begins with *creative hopelessness*, the realization that your old strategies for controlling your pain are not working and that it's time to try something new.

- The *Hexaflex* is the central model of ACT, outlining the six interconnected skills that build psychological flexibility: Acceptance, Defusion, Being Present, Self-as-Context, Values, and Committed Action.

- An ACT formulation of a problem focuses on how cognitive fusion and experiential avoidance are keeping a person stuck and disconnected from their values.

- The goal of the formulation is not to fix a person's thinking, but to identify the skills they need to build in order to live a more flexible and value-driven life.

This framework gives us leverage to move forward. We now have a clear model for how ACT works in practice. We've seen how it reframes a person's struggles and sets a new direction for therapy. With this understanding in place, we are ready to explore the specific, hands-on techniques that are used to build each of the six core skills of the Hexaflex.

Chapter 6: The ACT Toolkit

A Clinician's Guide to Core Techniques

We've explored the philosophy of ACT and seen how it can be used to understand a person's struggles in a new way. Now, we get to the most practical part: the tools themselves. This chapter is your hands-on guide to the core techniques of ACT. These are not just interesting ideas; they are simple, powerful exercises that you can start using right away to build psychological flexibility.

Think of this chapter as a workshop. We're going to roll up our sleeves and learn how to use the tools that bring the six core processes of the Hexaflex to life. We'll cover techniques for anchoring yourself in the present moment, for unhooking from difficult thoughts, for discovering what truly matters to you, and for turning those values into action. These exercises might feel a little strange or different at first, and that's perfectly okay. The goal is not to do them perfectly, but to practice them with an attitude of curiosity and openness. Let's begin.

Mindfulness and Present-Moment Awareness

The foundation of many ACT techniques is *mindfulness*. Mindfulness is simply the act of **paying attention to the present moment, on purpose, without judgment**. So much of our suffering happens when we are lost in our heads, worrying about the future or ruminating about the past. Mindfulness exercises are designed to gently guide our attention back to the here and now, which is the only place we can ever truly live our lives.

Simple Mindfulness Exercise: The Mindful Breath

This is one of the most basic and accessible mindfulness exercises. You can do it anywhere, for any length of time.

1. **Find a comfortable position.** You can be sitting, standing, or lying down. You can close your eyes or keep them open with a soft gaze.

2. **Bring your attention to your breath.** Notice the physical sensation of the air moving in and out of your body. You might feel it at your nostrils, in your chest, or in the rise and fall of your belly.

3. **Just notice.** You don't need to change your breathing in any way. Your only job is to observe the natural rhythm of your breath, moment by moment.

4. **When your mind wanders, gently guide it back.** And it *will* wander. That's what minds do. When you notice that your attention has drifted to a thought, a sound, or a sensation, just gently and kindly acknowledge where it went, and then guide it back to your breath.

The point of this exercise is not to stop your thoughts or to have a perfectly clear mind. The point is the act of noticing that you've wandered and gently coming back. Every time you do that, you are strengthening your "attention muscle."

Cognitive Defusion Techniques

Cognitive defusion is the art of unhooking from your thoughts. These techniques are designed to help you see your thoughts as what they are—just words and pictures—instead of getting caught up in their content. The goal is to create some space between you and your thoughts, so they have less influence over your actions. Defusion techniques are often playful and creative.

Here are a few popular defusion techniques:

1. "I'm Having the Thought That..."

This is a simple but powerful way to change your relationship with a thought. When a difficult thought shows up, instead of just thinking it, you rephrase it in your mind.

- Instead of thinking, "I'm a failure," you say to yourself, **"I'm having the thought that I'm a failure."**

- Instead of, "This anxiety will never end," you say, **"I'm noticing that my mind is telling me the story that this anxiety will never end."**

This small shift in language creates a bit of distance. It reminds you that you are not your thought; you are the one who is *noticing* the thought.

2. Thanking Your Mind

Your mind is not your enemy. It's an amazing problem-solving machine that is constantly trying to keep you safe. The problem is, it's often overzealous, seeing threats where there are none. This technique involves acknowledging your mind's efforts with a bit of gratitude and humor.

- When a worried thought pops up, like "What if you mess up the presentation?", you can say to yourself, **"Thanks, mind! I appreciate you trying to protect me from failure. I've got this."**

This changes the dynamic from a fight to a friendly conversation. You're not arguing with the thought; you're just acknowledging it and choosing not to get hooked by it.

3. Leaves on a Stream

This is a classic visualization exercise.

1. Find a comfortable place to sit and close your eyes.

2. Imagine yourself sitting by a gently flowing stream. There are leaves of all shapes and sizes floating by on the surface of the water.

3. For the next few minutes, your task is to place each thought that comes into your mind onto one of the leaves and watch it float away down the stream.

4. It doesn't matter if the thoughts are good or bad, happy or sad. Just place each one on a leaf and let it go. If you find yourself getting distracted or pulled into a thought, just notice that, and then gently place that thought on a leaf as well.

This exercise helps you practice the skill of letting your thoughts come and go without holding on to them.

Values Clarification Exercises

Getting clear on your values is like turning on the lights in a dark room. It gives you direction and purpose. These exercises are designed to help you connect with what truly matters to you.

The "Eulogy" Exercise

This exercise can feel a bit strange, but it's one of the most powerful ways to get in touch with your values.

1. Imagine that you are at your own funeral (or 80th birthday party, if that feels more comfortable). Someone who knows you very well is about to give a speech about your life.

2. Take a few minutes to write down what you would want them to say. What qualities would you want them to highlight? What would you want to be remembered for? How would you want to have treated yourself and others?

3. The words you write down—like "kind," "brave," "creative," "loving," "adventurous"—are clues to your deepest values.

The "Bull's-Eye" Exercise

This is a visual tool to help you assess how closely you are living in line with your values right now.

1. Draw a large target with four quadrants. Label the quadrants with four important life domains, such as "Work/Education," "Relationships," "Personal Growth/Health," and "Leisure."

2. In each quadrant, take a moment to think about your values. For example, in "Relationships," your values might be to be supportive, present, and loving.

3. Now, place an "X" in each quadrant to represent how much you have been living by those values recently. If you've been living fully in line with your values, place the X in the bull's-eye. If you've been living far away from your values, place it on the outer rings.

This is not an exercise in judgment. It's just an honest assessment that can help you see where you might want to focus your energy.

Committed Action

Values are just words until you put them into action. *Committed action* is about taking small, concrete steps that move you in the direction of your values. The key is to start small and focus on what you can do right now.

Setting Value-Driven Goals

1. **Pick a value.** Choose one of the values you identified in the previous exercises (e.g., "to be a more connected friend").

2. **Set a small, concrete goal.** What is one small action you could take in the next week that would move you in the direction of that value? It should be something specific and achievable. For example, "I will call my friend on Wednesday just to see how they are doing."

3. **Anticipate the barriers.** What difficult thoughts or feelings might show up and get in the way? (e.g., "I'm too busy," "They probably don't want to hear from me," the feeling of social anxiety).

47

4. **Make a plan.** How will you make room for those barriers and take the action anyway? (e.g., "When I have the thought that I'm too busy, I will thank my mind and remind myself that this is important to me. I will allow the feeling of anxiety to be there while I dial the number.")

This process connects your daily actions to your deepest sense of purpose, which is the heart of living a meaningful life.

Your Toolkit for a Valued Life

- *Mindfulness exercises*, like focusing on your breath, are about training your attention to stay in the present moment, which is where your life happens.

- *Cognitive defusion techniques* help you unhook from difficult thoughts by changing your relationship with them. You learn to see them as just thoughts, not as commands or truths.

- *Values clarification exercises* are tools to help you discover what you want your life to be about. Your values provide the direction and motivation for your journey.

- *Committed action* is about turning your values into concrete behaviors. You set small, value-driven goals and take action, even when it's uncomfortable.

You now have a set of practical skills for building psychological flexibility. We have explored the worlds of both I-CBT and ACT, seeing their different philosophies, formulations, and techniques. This sets the stage for our next section, where we will put these two powerful therapies side-by-side for a direct comparison, helping you to understand their fundamental differences and decide which path might be right for you.

Chapter 7: Philosophical Underpinnings — Truth vs. Workability

When you get right down to it, every approach to therapy is built on a set of core beliefs about what causes human suffering and what helps people get better. These are the deep, philosophical foundations that shape everything else—the techniques, the goals, and the way a therapist interacts with you. So far, we've looked at the practical tools of I-CBT and ACT. Now, it's time to go a little deeper and explore the fundamental ideas that make these two therapies so different from each other.

Understanding these core philosophies is incredibly important. It's like knowing the difference between the architectural principles of a skyscraper and a suspension bridge. Both are amazing structures, but they are built on entirely different ideas about how to handle stress and pressure. In this chapter, we're going to compare the philosophical underpinnings of I-CBT and ACT. We'll look at how they take completely opposite stances on the nature of thoughts, the definition of reality, and the role of anxiety in our lives. This comparison will help you understand not just *what* you do in these therapies, but *why* you do it.

The Stance on Thoughts

The most fundamental difference between I-CBT and ACT lies in how they view your thoughts. When a difficult, obsessive thought shows up, what should you do with it? The answer to this question reveals the core philosophy of each approach.

I-CBT: The Quest for Truth and Logical Validity

I-CBT is deeply invested in the question of whether a thought is **true**. More specifically, it is concerned with the *logical validity* of the reasoning process that produced the thought. From an I-CBT perspective, an obsessional doubt is not just a random mental event; it is a faulty conclusion that has been reached through a flawed process of thinking. As researchers from Weston Family Psychology explain, I-CBT views obsessions as the result of a reasoning story that relies too much on imagination and not enough on what your senses are telling you.

The entire therapeutic process in I-CBT is designed to act like a logical investigation. You are taught to put your obsessional doubt on trial and examine the evidence. The goal is to prove, beyond a reasonable doubt, that the thought is invalid because the reasoning behind it is unsound. You learn to see that the doubt is not based on the facts of the present moment but on a fictional narrative.

Let's say you have the thought, "I might have hit someone with my car."

- **I-CBT asks: Is this a valid conclusion?** It would guide you to examine the reasoning. "Did I feel a bump? Did I hear a noise? Did I see anything in my mirrors? No. My senses are telling me nothing happened. Therefore, the thought that I *might* have hit someone is a product of a faulty reasoning process, not reality. The conclusion is false."

The goal here is to achieve a genuine resolution of the doubt. By dismantling the faulty logic, you arrive at the truth of the situation, and the doubt dissolves.

ACT: The Focus on Workability

ACT, on the other hand, is not at all interested in whether a thought is true or false. Instead, it asks a completely different question: **Is getting entangled with this thought *workable*?** In other words, is

51

paying attention to this thought, arguing with it, and letting it guide your actions helping you move toward the life you want to live?

From an ACT perspective, trying to figure out if a thought is true is often a trap. Our minds can generate an endless supply of thoughts, and trying to win a debate with your own mind is an exhausting and unwinnable game. According to Steven Hayes and his colleagues who developed ACT, the problem isn't the thought itself, but our fusion with it—the way we get hooked by it and treat it as an absolute truth.

Let's go back to the thought, "I might have hit someone with my car."

- **ACT asks: Is it helpful to get into a debate with this thought?** It would guide you to notice the thought without getting hooked. "Ah, there's the 'hit-and-run story' again. I notice my mind is offering me this thought. Is it workable for me to spend the next hour ruminating about this and driving back to check? Or would it be more workable to thank my mind for trying to keep me safe and then put my attention back on driving home to my family?"

The goal in ACT is not to prove the thought false, but to make it *irrelevant*. You learn to see it as just a thought, a bit of mental noise, and you choose to put your energy into your actions and your values instead. The question is never "Is it true?" but always "Is it helpful?".

Reflection: Think of a recent worry. Did you spend more time trying to figure out if it was true, or did you notice how much energy you were losing by getting stuck on it? Which question—"Is it true?" or "Is it workable?"—feels more empowering to you right now?

The Approach to Reality

This difference in how the two therapies treat thoughts leads to a very different approach to the concept of reality itself. Both therapies want to help you live in the "real world," but they define that world in very different ways.

I-CBT: Re-establishing Trust in Objective, Sensory Reality

The core mission of I-CBT is to help you rebuild your trust in the objective, physical, sensory world. The problem in obsessive thinking, according to I-CBT, is that you have lost contact with this reality. You have started to believe that the imaginary world inside your head is more real and more reliable than what your own five senses are telling you. This is the essence of what is called "inferential confusion."

The techniques in I-CBT, like the reality-sensing exercises we discussed, are all designed to pull you out of the fictional narrative and ground you back in the physical world. The therapy teaches you to privilege the data you get from your senses—what you can see, hear, touch, taste, and smell—over the "what if" scenarios generated by your imagination. As described by the clinicians at Anxiety Specialists of St. Louis, I-CBT helps you learn to make evidence-based conclusions that are grounded in real life, not in imagination.

The goal is to restore your faith in your own ability to perceive reality accurately. It's about learning to trust that if you see the stove is off, it is off, and that this sensory fact is more trustworthy than the imaginary story about a potential fire.

ACT: Accepting Your Internal Reality as It Is

ACT takes a different approach. It agrees that it's important to be in contact with the present moment, but it defines that present moment as including *both* your external and your internal reality. Your internal reality consists of your thoughts, feelings, memories, and physical sensations.

From an ACT perspective, trying to fight or get rid of your internal reality is a fool's errand. Your thoughts and feelings are what they are. They are part of your experience in this moment. The goal of ACT is not to replace your internal reality with a more "objective" one, but to learn how to **accept your internal reality just as it is, without judgment and without a struggle**.

This is a key point. ACT doesn't ask you to believe your thoughts are true. It just asks you to acknowledge that they are *there*. They are part of your inner landscape in this moment. The goal is to stop the war with your own mind and to make peace with the fact that your inner world will sometimes be uncomfortable. As explained in an article from The Chelsea Psychology Clinic, ACT encourages you to move closer to difficult feelings rather than trying to push them away.

So, while I-CBT helps you ground yourself in the external world to prove your internal doubts are false, ACT helps you ground yourself in the present moment as a whole, allowing your internal experiences to be there without letting them control you.

The Role of Anxiety

Finally, the two therapies have fundamentally different views on the role of anxiety. Is anxiety the primary problem to be solved, or is it a normal part of life to be accepted?

I-CBT: Anxiety as a Secondary Problem to Be Eliminated

In the I-CBT model, anxiety is seen as a **secondary problem**. It is a byproduct of the primary problem, which is the faulty reasoning process that creates the obsessional doubt. The logic is simple and linear: first comes the flawed reasoning, which leads to an invalid doubt, and it is this doubt that then triggers the feeling of anxiety.

Therefore, the goal of I-CBT is to **eliminate the anxiety by resolving the doubt that causes it**. The therapy doesn't focus on teaching you how to tolerate anxiety. It focuses on showing you that, based on the evidence of reality, there is no valid reason for the anxiety to exist in the first place. According to research published in the journal *Psychotherapy and Psychosomatics*, I-CBT is hypothesized to not provoke high levels of anxiety because it works "upstream" to address the source of the doubt.

If you successfully dismantle the obsessional narrative and see that the doubt is based on fiction, the logical foundation for the anxiety crumbles. The anxiety simply dissolves because its reason for being there is gone.

ACT: Anxiety as an Inevitable Part of a Valued Life

ACT, on the other hand, views anxiety and other forms of discomfort as **an inevitable and normal part of being human**. The goal is not to eliminate anxiety. The goal is to learn how to live a full and meaningful life even when anxiety shows up.

From an ACT perspective, a life without any anxiety would be a very small life. To do anything that truly matters to you—whether it's asking someone on a date, giving a presentation, or being a vulnerable and loving parent—you will inevitably feel some anxiety. If you make it your life's mission to never feel anxious, you will have to give up on most of the things you care about.

Therefore, ACT teaches you to **accept anxiety as a companion that will sometimes show up on your journey**. You learn to make room for it, to let it be there in your body, without letting it stop you from taking action in the direction of your values. As described by the experts at Talkspace, ACT teaches you to sit in discomfort if it serves a valuable purpose. The goal is not to feel less anxiety, but to be less controlled by it.

Two Different Worlds

- **On Thoughts:** I-CBT is a truth-focused therapy that asks, "Is this thought valid?" It aims to dismantle faulty reasoning. ACT is a workability-focused therapy that asks, "Is getting hooked by this thought helpful?" It aims to make the thought irrelevant.

- **On Reality:** I-CBT's goal is to rebuild your trust in the objective, sensory world as the ultimate source of truth. ACT's goal is to help you accept your entire present-moment experience—both internal and external—without a struggle.

- **On Anxiety:** I-CBT sees anxiety as a secondary problem that can be eliminated by resolving the primary doubt. ACT sees anxiety as a normal part of life that should be accepted in the service of living according to your values.

This foundation creates room for the next part of our discussion. Now that we have a clear understanding of the deep philosophical differences between these two approaches, we can explore how these differences translate into the practical experience of therapy. In the next chapter, we will look at how I-CBT and ACT work in the real world, comparing their mechanisms of change, the role of the therapist, and the kinds of homework you can expect.

Chapter 8: Mechanisms of Change and The Clinician's Stance

When you decide to start therapy, you're not just choosing a set of techniques; you're entering into a process and a relationship. How does change actually happen in therapy? What is the therapist's job, and what is yours? The answers to these questions can look very different depending on the approach being used. The philosophical differences between I-CBT and ACT that we just explored naturally lead to very different ways of working in the therapy room.

This chapter is about the practical realities of what it's like to be in I-CBT versus ACT. We'll compare how each therapy believes change occurs, what you can expect from your therapist, and the kind of work you'll be asked to do between sessions. Think of this as a behind-the-scenes tour of the two approaches. By understanding these practical differences, you'll be in a much better position to know which style of working might be the best fit for you and your personality.

How They Work

At the most basic level, how do these therapies actually help people get better? What is the engine of change in each model? While both aim to free you from the grip of obsessional thinking, they go about it in fundamentally different ways.

I-CBT: Change Through Cognitive Insight and Reasoning

The mechanism of change in I-CBT is primarily **cognitive**. Change happens when you have a series of "aha!" moments—insights into the faulty logic that has been driving your obsessive doubts. It's a process of education and discovery. You learn to see the "trick" behind your OCD, and once you see it, it loses its power.

As we discussed earlier, I-CBT is an "upstream" intervention. It targets the very beginning of the obsessional sequence. The theory, as outlined in a clinical trial registered on ClinicalTrials.gov, is that if you can change the reasoning that leads to the initial doubt, you will logically and necessarily eliminate all the downstream consequences, like anxiety and compulsions.

The process works like this:

1. **You learn the theory:** You are taught the I-CBT model of how obsessional doubts are created through inferential confusion.

2. **You apply it to yourself:** You work to identify your own obsessional narrative, your feared self, and the specific reasoning errors you make.

3. **You have a realization:** Through this process, you come to a deep, personal understanding that your doubt is not based on reality. It's not just an intellectual idea; it's a felt sense of clarity. One user on Reddit described this realization as a feeling of lightness and an "of course that's how it works!" moment.

4. **The doubt dissolves:** Once you truly see the doubt as an irrelevant product of a faulty process, it loses its believability and its emotional punch.

In I-CBT, the "knowing" comes before the "doing." You gain a new understanding first, and that new understanding is what allows you to change your behavior (i.e., to stop performing compulsions).

ACT: Change Through Behavioral Experience and Context

The mechanism of change in ACT is primarily **behavioral**. Change doesn't happen because you think your way out of a problem; it happens because you *act* your way into a new way of living. It's a process of learning through direct experience.

ACT is not focused on changing the content of your thoughts. Instead, it focuses on changing the *context* in which your thoughts occur. By using mindfulness and defusion techniques, you learn to hold your thoughts more lightly. You change your relationship to them. This creates a space where you can choose your actions based on your values, rather than reacting automatically to your thoughts and feelings.

The process looks more like this:

1. **You clarify your values:** You get clear on what you want your life to be about.

2. **You practice acceptance and defusion:** You learn skills to make room for discomfort and to unhook from unhelpful thoughts.

3. **You take committed action:** You start taking small, deliberate steps in the direction of your values, even if it's scary.

4. **You learn from experience:** As you take these actions, you learn through direct experience that you *can* move toward what matters to you, even when your mind is telling you scary stories. You learn that your thoughts don't have to control you.

In ACT, the "doing" comes before the "knowing." You change your behavior first, and that new behavior is what teaches you that you are more than your thoughts and that you can handle more than you think.

The Therapist's Role

The role of the therapist is also quite different in these two approaches. While any good therapist will be warm, empathetic, and non-judgmental, their specific job in the session will vary depending on the model they are using.

The I-CBT Therapist: The Collaborative Detective and Teacher

In I-CBT, the therapist takes on the role of a **collaborative detective and a teacher**. They are an expert on the I-CBT model, and their job is to teach it to you and then help you apply it to your own life.

- **As a teacher,** the therapist will explain the concepts of inferential confusion, the obsessional narrative, and the feared self. They will use clear language, metaphors, and diagrams to help you understand the theory. As described in a training course offered by Catherine Goldhouse, a good I-CBT therapist needs to be a good teacher who can explain things in a variety of ways.

- **As a detective,** the therapist will work with you to uncover the specific details of your faulty reasoning. They will ask a lot of questions to help you map out your narrative and identify the exact moments where you slip from reality into imagination. They are your partner in the investigation, helping you find the clues that will solve the mystery of your OCD.

The relationship is collaborative, but there is a clear sense that the therapist is guiding you through a structured learning process.

The ACT Therapist: The Compassionate Coach and Guide

In ACT, the therapist's role is more like that of a **compassionate coach and guide**. They are not there to teach you a set of facts, but to help you connect with your own experience and your own wisdom.

- **As a coach,** the therapist will encourage you, challenge you, and support you as you take the difficult steps of facing your discomfort and moving toward your values. They are on the sidelines, cheering you on as you learn to live a more flexible life.

- **As a guide,** the therapist will lead you through experiential exercises, like mindfulness meditations and defusion techniques. They are not just talking *about* these concepts; they are helping you *experience* them directly in the session. The therapist is a fellow traveler on the journey, modeling acceptance and compassion for their own inner experience as well as for yours.

The stance is less about being an expert who has the answers and more about being a guide who can help you find your own answers. The relationship is deeply human and is itself a model for the kind of open, aware, and engaged life that ACT promotes.

Use of Homework

Finally, the work you do between sessions—often called homework—looks quite different in the two therapies. In both models, this work is considered essential for progress.

I-CBT Homework

Structured Skill-Building

The homework in I-CBT is typically very **structured and focused on building specific cognitive skills**. It's like doing exercises from a textbook to reinforce what you learned in class.

You might be asked to:

- Keep a log of your obsessional doubts and practice differentiating them from normal doubts.

- Write out your full obsessional narrative for a specific theme.

- Practice reality-sensing exercises when you notice a doubt and record your experience.

- Complete worksheets that help you identify your feared self and gather evidence for your real self.

The homework is designed to help you internalize the I-CBT model and get better at applying the reasoning skills in your daily life. According to information from the International OCD Foundation, practicing the skills you learn in therapy between sessions is a key part of the I-CBT process.

ACT Homework: Value-Driven Behavioral Experiments

The homework in ACT is more like a series of **behavioral experiments that are guided by your values**. It's less about worksheets and more about getting out into your life and trying new things.

You might be asked to:

- Practice a short mindfulness exercise every day.

- Identify one small action you can take this week that is in line with one of your core values, and then do it.

- Notice when you get fused with a particular thought and practice a defusion technique.

- Willingly expose yourself to a situation you've been avoiding, not to get rid of anxiety, but to practice being the person you want to be.

The homework is designed to be experiential. It's about learning by doing and building a life that matters to you, one small, committed action at a time.

Different Ways of Working

- **How They Work:** I-CBT creates change through cognitive insight; you learn your way into a new way of acting. ACT creates change through behavioral experience; you act your way into a new way of knowing.

- **The Therapist's Role:** The I-CBT therapist is a teacher and a detective, guiding you through a structured learning process. The ACT therapist is a coach and a guide, helping you connect with your own experience.

- **Use of Homework:** I-CBT homework involves structured, skill-building exercises to help you master the cognitive model. ACT homework involves value-driven behavioral experiments to help you build a more meaningful life.

We can see that I-CBT and ACT are not just different in their techniques, but in their entire way of working. They offer two distinct paths, each with its own unique style and process. This understanding is crucial as we move into the final part of our comparison, where we will discuss how to choose the right path for you and explore the exciting possibility of integrating these two powerful approaches.

Chapter 9: A Clinician's Decision Guide: When to Dismantle, When to Defuse

We've now explored the worlds of I-CBT and ACT in detail. We've seen their different philosophies, their unique toolkits, and the different ways they approach the process of therapy. This naturally leads to a very practical question: How do you choose? When you're sitting with a difficult thought, is it better to dismantle it with logic or to defuse from it with mindfulness? Which path is the right one for you?

The truth is, there is no single "best" approach for everyone. The most effective therapy is often the one that best fits your personality, your goals, and the specific nature of your struggles. This chapter is designed to be a practical guide to help you make that choice. We'll look at the specific signs and symptoms that might suggest one approach would be a better fit than the other. We'll also provide a simple decision-making tool to help you think through your options. This isn't about finding a perfect answer, but about making an informed and empowered choice on your journey toward a freer and more meaningful life.

Assessing Client Suitability

Just as a doctor wouldn't prescribe the same medicine for every illness, a good therapist doesn't use a one-size-fits-all approach. Different people respond to different kinds of therapy. Let's look at some of the key factors that might make I-CBT or ACT a particularly good fit for someone.

Indications for I-CBT

I-CBT, with its focus on logic, reasoning, and evidence, tends to be a very good match for people with certain presentations and preferences.

- **People with poor insight or overvalued ideation.** This is a clinical way of saying that someone is very, very convinced that their obsessive fears are real. They don't just have a nagging doubt; they have a deeply held belief that feels like a fact. For these individuals, therapies that ask them to simply tolerate their anxiety can feel invalidating or even impossible. I-CBT is uniquely suited for this because it doesn't ask you to tolerate the fear; it helps you investigate the belief itself. In fact, a large randomized controlled trial found that while I-CBT was as effective as standard CBT overall, it was significantly more effective for the subgroup of patients with high levels of overvalued ideation.

- **A preference for a logical, reasoning-based approach.** Some people are naturally analytical. They like to understand *why* things work the way they do. They want a clear, step-by-step process for solving a problem. For these individuals, the structured, educational, and detective-like nature of I-CBT can be very appealing. It provides a clear framework and a set of logical tools that can feel very empowering.

- **A history of ERP refusal or failure.** Exposure and Response Prevention (ERP) is the gold-standard treatment for OCD, but it can be very challenging. It requires a willingness to face your worst fears head-on, which can generate a great deal of anxiety. Research has shown that a significant number of people either refuse to start ERP or drop out of treatment because the distress is too high. I-CBT offers a powerful, evidence-based alternative that does not require this high level of anxiety. For anyone who has found ERP to be too difficult or who is hesitant to try it, I-CBT is an excellent option to consider.

Indications for ACT

ACT, with its emphasis on acceptance, mindfulness, and values, is often a great fit for people who are looking for a more holistic and life-affirming approach.

- **People struggling with broad experiential avoidance.** Some people's struggles aren't limited to one specific fear. They find themselves in a constant battle with a wide range of uncomfortable thoughts and feelings. They may have spent years trying to control their anxiety, sadness, or self-doubt, only to find that their lives have become smaller and more restricted. ACT is designed for this exact problem. It directly targets the pattern of experiential avoidance and teaches a new way of relating to all internal experiences.

- **A desire for a holistic, values-based approach.** Some people come to therapy not just to get rid of a symptom, but to build a better life. They are asking bigger questions about purpose, meaning, and what they want to stand for. ACT is perfectly suited for this, as it places your personal values at the very center of the therapeutic process. The goal isn't just to feel better; it's to live better, in a way that is deeply aligned with what matters to you.

- **Dealing with chronic conditions where distress is unavoidable.** ACT has been shown to be particularly helpful for people dealing with situations where some level of pain or discomfort is a long-term reality, such as chronic pain, chronic illness, or ongoing life stressors. In these situations, a therapy that promises to eliminate distress can feel unrealistic. ACT offers a more compassionate and workable approach: it teaches you how to live a rich and meaningful life *alongside* your pain, rather than putting your life on hold until the pain goes away.

Reflection: As you read through these descriptions, which one resonates more with you? Do you see yourself more in the I-CBT profile or the ACT profile? What does your gut tell you about which approach might be a better fit for your personality and your goals?

A Decision-Making Tree

To help you think through this choice more systematically, here is a simple decision-making tree. Start at the top and follow the path that best describes your situation. This is not a scientific diagnostic tool, but rather a guide to help you clarify your own thinking.

Start Here: What is my primary goal in seeking help?

1. **"My main goal is to understand and resolve a specific, looping doubt that I am convinced is true. I want to prove to myself that my fear is not based in reality."**

   o This points toward **I-CBT**. Your focus is on the *truth* and *validity* of a specific thought process. You are looking for a logical resolution.

2. **"My main goal is to stop being controlled by a wide range of uncomfortable thoughts and feelings. I want to learn how to live a full life, even when I feel anxious or sad."**

   o This points toward **ACT**. Your focus is on changing your *relationship* with your internal experiences and living a life guided by your values.

If you chose #1 (leaning toward I-CBT), ask yourself this:

- **Do I enjoy structured, logical, and educational approaches to problem-solving?**

   o If **yes**, this strengthens the case for **I-CBT**.

   o If **no**, you might still benefit from I-CBT, but you could also consider if the values-based approach of ACT might be a better fit for your style.

67

If you chose #2 (leaning toward ACT), ask yourself this:

- **Am I more interested in building a meaningful life than in getting rid of my anxiety?**

    ○ If **yes**, this strengthens the case for **ACT**.

    ○ If **no**, and your primary goal is symptom reduction, you might find the direct, problem-solving approach of I-CBT to be more appealing.

Final Consideration for Everyone:

- **Have I tried Exposure and Response Prevention (ERP) before and found it too difficult or ineffective?**

    ○ If **yes**, then **I-CBT** is a particularly strong alternative to consider, as it is an evidence-based treatment for OCD that does not rely on exposure.

By walking through these questions, you can get a clearer sense of which therapeutic philosophy and style of working might be the best starting point for you.

Choosing Your Path

- **When to consider I-CBT:** This approach may be particularly well-suited for you if you have a very strong conviction in your obsessive fears, if you prefer a logical and structured approach, or if you have been unable or unwilling to engage in exposure-based therapies like ERP.

- **When to consider ACT:** This approach may be a great fit if you struggle with a broad pattern of avoiding discomfort, if you are seeking a more holistic and values-based way of living, or if you are dealing with chronic conditions where some level of distress is unavoidable.

- **A decision-making tool** can help you clarify your own goals and preferences, guiding you toward the approach that is most aligned with what you are looking for in therapy.

These building blocks enable us to consider an even more flexible approach. What if the choice isn't about picking one therapy over the other? What if you could get the best of both worlds? In the next chapter, we will explore the exciting possibilities of an integrative approach, looking at how the tools of I-CBT and ACT can be blended together to create a truly personalized path to recovery.

Chapter 10: An Integrative Approach

So far, we've been treating I-CBT and ACT as two separate paths, each with its own map and its own destination. But what if they aren't mutually exclusive? What if, instead of choosing one road, you could build a bridge between them? In the world of modern therapy, more and more clinicians are realizing that the most effective approach is often an integrative one—one that thoughtfully combines the best tools from different models to meet the unique needs of each person.

This chapter is about building that bridge. We'll explore the exciting potential of blending I-CBT and ACT. We'll look at how you might use the two therapies at different stages of your recovery, and how specific techniques from one can actually enhance the other. This is where therapy becomes less of a rigid protocol and more of a creative art. It's about moving beyond the question of "Dismantle or Defuse?" and starting to ask, "When is it helpful to dismantle, and when is it helpful to defuse?"

Blending Modalities

One of the most straightforward ways to integrate I-CBT and ACT is to use them at different points in the therapeutic journey. Each therapy has strengths that may be particularly useful at different stages of recovery.

A common and effective way to blend them is to start with a more structured, symptom-focused approach and then move toward a broader, more values-based way of living. As described by the therapists at The Chelsea Psychology Clinic, it's possible to begin with a CBT-style approach to stabilize acute symptoms and then transition to ACT for long-term resilience.

Here's what that might look like:

- **Phase 1: Using I-CBT for Acute Symptom Stabilization.**
  When you are in the thick of an obsessive-compulsive cycle,
  it can feel like you are drowning. Your primary goal is to get
  your head above water. I-CBT is exceptionally good for this.
  Its structured, logical approach can provide a sense of safety
  and control. By learning to deconstruct your obsessional
  narrative and see the faulty reasoning behind your doubts, you
  can significantly reduce the intensity and frequency of your
  symptoms. This is the "dismantling" phase, where you take
  apart the machine of OCD so it no longer runs your life.

- **Phase 2: Using ACT for Long-Term Resilience and Value-
  Driven Living.** Once your acute symptoms have stabilized
  and you're no longer drowning in doubt, a new question often
  arises: "Now what?" You've gotten rid of the problem, but
  what do you want to build in its place? This is where ACT can
  be incredibly powerful. After you've cleared the ground with
  I-CBT, you can use the tools of ACT to build a rich,
  meaningful, and resilient life. You can clarify your values,
  practice accepting the normal ups and downs of life, and
  commit to taking action in the service of what matters most to
  you. This is the "defusing" and "doing" phase, where you
  learn to navigate the rest of your life with flexibility and
  purpose.

This two-phase approach gives you the best of both worlds. You get
the targeted, problem-solving power of I-CBT when you need it most,
and the broad, life-enhancing wisdom of ACT to guide you in the long
run.

Using I-CBT Techniques to Enhance ACT

Even if you are primarily using an ACT approach, you can borrow
specific techniques from I-CBT to make your ACT work even more
powerful. The two therapies can complement each other in surprising
ways.

How deconstructing an obsessional narrative can serve as a powerful defusion exercise.

In ACT, the goal of cognitive defusion is to create distance from your thoughts—to see them as just stories, not as literal truths. One of the most effective ways to see that something is a story is to take it apart and look at how it was constructed. This is exactly what you do in I-CBT when you deconstruct an obsessional narrative.

Imagine you are working with the thought, "I am a contaminated person."

- A standard **ACT** defusion technique might be to say, "I'm having the thought that I am a contaminated person."

- An **I-CBT-enhanced** defusion technique would be to actually map out the story. You could say, "Ah, there's the 'contaminated person' story. I notice it's made up of a memory of being sick once, a news article I read about germs, and a lot of 'what if' thoughts. It's just a collection of mental bits and pieces that my mind has stitched together."

By deconstructing the narrative in this way, you are doing more than just labeling the thought; you are seeing its fictional nature from the inside out. This can be an incredibly powerful way to defuse from the story and rob it of its believability. You're not just seeing that it's a story; you're seeing *how* it's a story.

Using ACT Techniques to Enhance I-CBT

The bridge between these two therapies runs in both directions. If you are primarily using an I-CBT approach, you can borrow tools from ACT to help you navigate the process more effectively.

How mindfulness and acceptance can help you tolerate the process of engaging with your faulty reasoning without resorting to compulsions.

The process of I-CBT, while not as anxiety-provoking as ERP, can still be uncomfortable. When you start to investigate your obsessional doubts, you are deliberately bringing your attention to the very thoughts that cause you distress. In these moments, you might feel a strong urge to perform a compulsion to get rid of the discomfort.

This is where the ACT skills of mindfulness and acceptance can be incredibly helpful.

- **Mindfulness** can help you stay grounded and present as you do the cognitive work of I-CBT. You can learn to notice the urge to perform a compulsion as just a sensation in your body, without having to act on it.

- **Acceptance** can help you make room for the anxiety that might arise during the process. You can learn to allow the feeling of doubt or uncertainty to be there, without struggling against it, while you continue to do the logical work of examining your reasoning.

By using these ACT skills, you can create a safe and stable inner space from which to do the challenging work of I-CBT. You're using acceptance to help you tolerate the short-term discomfort of the dismantling process, which makes that process much more manageable and effective.

Reflection: Think about a time you felt a strong urge to do something compulsive (like check something, ask for reassurance, or avoid a situation). What would it have been like to just notice that urge as a physical sensation, without judging it or needing to act on it? This is the kind of skill that ACT can bring to any therapeutic approach.

The Best of Both Worlds

- **Blending Modalities:** It is possible to use I-CBT and ACT at different stages of therapy. You might use I-CBT first to stabilize acute symptoms and then transition to ACT to build long-term resilience and a value-driven life.

- **Enhancing ACT with I-CBT:** The I-CBT technique of deconstructing an obsessional narrative can be used as a powerful cognitive defusion exercise, helping you to see your thoughts as the fictional stories they are.

- **Enhancing I-CBT with ACT:** The ACT skills of mindfulness and acceptance can help you tolerate the discomfort of investigating your faulty reasoning, making the I-CBT process more manageable and effective.

- An integrative approach allows for a flexible, personalized therapy that can be tailored to your unique needs at every stage of your journey.

This flexibility opens up a world of possibilities. It shows that these powerful therapies don't have to be confined to their original boxes. As we will see in the next chapter, the core principles of both I-CBT and ACT can be applied to a wide range of human struggles, far beyond the specific problem of OCD.

Chapter 11: Applying the Models to Other Presentations

While I-CBT was originally developed specifically for Obsessive-Compulsive Disorder, and ACT is known for its broad applicability, the core principles of both therapies have a reach that extends far beyond any single diagnosis. The human mind, after all, tends to get stuck in similar ways, regardless of the specific content of our worries. The patterns of faulty reasoning, getting hooked by thoughts, and avoiding discomfort are not unique to OCD. They show up in many different forms of psychological suffering.

This chapter is about expanding our view and seeing how the powerful tools of I-CBT and ACT can be applied to a wider range of common human problems. We'll look at how these models can be adapted to help with other anxiety disorders, the relentless pressure of perfectionism, and even the heavy weight of depression and chronic pain. By doing this, we can see that these therapies are not just about treating a disorder; they are about teaching fundamental skills for living a more sane, flexible, and meaningful life.

Anxiety Disorders

The core engines of anxiety—catastrophic thinking and avoidance—are prime targets for both I-CBT and ACT. Let's look at how each model would approach a few common anxiety disorders.

Social Anxiety

- **An I-CBT Approach:** Social anxiety is often driven by the inference of negative judgment from others, even when there is no evidence for it. An I-CBT approach would focus on the faulty reasoning that leads to the conclusion, "Everyone thinks I'm awkward." It would help you see that this is an inference based on an internal, imaginary story (your "feared self" as the socially inept person), not on the reality of the social situation. You would learn to trust your senses—what you can actually see and hear—rather than the internal narrative of judgment.

- **An ACT Approach:** An ACT approach would not debate whether people are judging you. Instead, it would focus on what you are avoiding. It would help you clarify your value of connection and then take committed action toward that value (e.g., going to a party), while practicing acceptance of the anxious feelings that show up. You would learn to let the thought "They think I'm awkward" be there, without letting it stop you from having a conversation.

Health Anxiety

- **An I-CBT Approach:** Health anxiety involves making catastrophic leaps from benign bodily sensations to serious illnesses. As described by the clinicians at Anxiety Specialists of St. Louis, an I-CBT approach would help you slow down and see the faulty reasoning that takes you from "a tingling in my foot" to "I must have multiple sclerosis." It would help you deconstruct the narrative, identify the feared self (e.g., "the vulnerable person who can't cope with illness"), and ground yourself in the simple, sensory reality of the moment.

- **An ACT Approach:** An ACT approach would focus on the unworkability of constantly seeking reassurance and checking your body. It would help you accept the presence of uncomfortable physical sensations and the uncertainty of health, while committing to actions that align with a value of vitality (e.g., exercising, eating well, and engaging in life, rather than spending hours on medical websites).

Perfectionism

Clinical perfectionism is the rigid belief that anything less than a perfect outcome is a catastrophic failure. It is a relentless and exhausting way to live, and both I-CBT and ACT offer powerful ways to address it.

- **An I-CBT Approach:** Perfectionism is fueled by a series of faulty inferences, such as, "If I make a small mistake on this report, my boss will think I'm incompetent and I will lose my job." An I-CBT approach would help you dismantle the reasoning behind this catastrophic conclusion. It would have you examine the evidence from your past experiences and the reality of your work environment to show that this inference is not logically sound. The goal is to prove that the equation "mistake = catastrophe" is false.

- **An ACT Approach:** An ACT approach would focus on the values that are being sacrificed in the pursuit of perfection (e.g., creativity, connection, well-being). It would help you accept the discomfort and anxiety that come with the possibility of making a mistake, so that you can pursue your valued goals. You would practice cognitive defusion with perfectionistic thoughts like, "This has to be perfect," seeing them as just thoughts, not commands. The goal is to learn to tolerate imperfection in the service of a richer, more engaged life. Research on internet-based CBT for perfectionism, such as the study by Alexander Rozental and his colleagues, has shown that these kinds of cognitive and behavioral strategies can be very effective. (Rozental,et al, 2017)

Depression and Chronic Pain

While we have focused primarily on anxiety-based problems, the principles of ACT, in particular, are incredibly well-suited for conditions like depression and chronic pain.

- **Depression:** Depression often involves deep fusion with negative self-judgments ("I'm worthless," "Things will never get better") and a withdrawal from life. An ACT approach is a natural fit here. It helps people defuse from these painful thoughts, accept the presence of low mood and low energy, and take small, committed actions in the direction of their values. This process of behavioral activation—doing what matters even when you don't feel like it—is one of the most powerful ways to break the cycle of depression.

- **Chronic Pain:** Chronic pain is a situation where the goal of eliminating discomfort is often unrealistic. This is where ACT truly shines. It helps people stop the exhausting and often fruitless struggle to get rid of their pain. Instead, it teaches them how to accept the presence of the pain and build a meaningful life *around* it. They learn to defuse from catastrophic thoughts about the pain, accept the physical sensations as they are, and redirect their energy from pain management to value-driven living.

By expanding our view, we can see that the skills taught in I-CBT and ACT are not just for one specific problem. They are fundamental life skills that can be applied to a wide range of human struggles, helping us to reason more clearly, to relate to our own minds with more flexibility, and to build lives of purpose and meaning.

A Wider Application

- **Anxiety Disorders:** The principles of I-CBT can be used to dismantle the faulty reasoning behind social and health anxieties, while ACT can help people accept their anxious feelings and take value-driven action.

- **Perfectionism:** I-CBT can challenge the catastrophic inference that "mistake = failure," while ACT can help people accept the discomfort of imperfection in order to live a more flexible and meaningful life.

- **Depression and Chronic Pain:** ACT is particularly well-suited for these conditions, as it helps people stop the struggle with their internal experiences and redirect their energy toward building a life that matters to them, even when pain is present.

- The core skills of these therapies are transdiagnostic, meaning they can be applied to the underlying processes that drive many different forms of psychological suffering.

We are now ready to bring our exploration to a close. We have discussed the theory, practice, and application of two of the most powerful modern therapies. In our conclusion, we will summarize the key distinctions of the "Dismantle vs. Defuse" framework and reflect on the future of a more personalized and effective approach to cognitive therapy.

Conclusion: The Future of Personalized Cognitive Therapy

We have traveled a long way together on this journey. We started by exploring the familiar landscape of cognitive therapy and then ventured into two newer, powerful, and very different territories: Inference-Based Cognitive Behavioral Therapy and Acceptance and Commitment Therapy. We've examined their core philosophies, learned their practical techniques, and seen how they can be applied to a wide range of human struggles. We've wrestled with the central question that has guided our exploration: When a difficult thought shows up, is it better to dismantle it or to defuse from it?

As we bring our journey to a close, it's time to zoom out and look at the bigger picture. In this final chapter, we will summarize the key distinctions between I-CBT and ACT, reflect on the importance of having a diverse toolkit for the mind, and look ahead to the exciting future of a more personalized and flexible approach to therapy. This isn't just the end of a book; it's the beginning of a new way of thinking about how we can all find more freedom and meaning in our lives.

Summary of Key Distinctions

At the heart of this book has been the "Dismantle vs. Defuse" framework. This simple phrase captures the profound philosophical and practical differences between I-CBT and ACT. Let's do a final review of these key distinctions.

- **The Stance on Thoughts:**
  - **I-CBT (Dismantle):** This approach is fundamentally concerned with the **truth and logical validity** of your thoughts. It teaches you to be a detective, to investigate the faulty reasoning process that creates an obsessional

80

doubt, and to prove that the doubt is not based in reality. The goal is to resolve the doubt by showing that it is a false conclusion.

- ○ **ACT (Defuse):** This approach is not concerned with the truth of your thoughts, but with their **workability**. It teaches you to be an observer, to notice your thoughts without getting hooked by them, and to ask whether getting entangled in them is helping you live the life you want. The goal is to make the thought irrelevant by changing your relationship to it.

- **The Approach to Reality:**

  - ○ **I-CBT:** The goal is to re-establish your trust in **objective, sensory reality**. It teaches you to privilege the evidence of your five senses over the imaginary stories in your head.

  - ○ **ACT:** The goal is to learn to accept your **entire present-moment experience**, including your internal reality of thoughts and feelings, without a struggle.

- **The Role of Anxiety:**

  - ○ **I-CBT:** Anxiety is seen as a **secondary problem** that is caused by the primary doubt. The goal is to eliminate the anxiety by resolving the doubt.

  - ○ **ACT:** Anxiety is seen as a **normal and inevitable part of life**. The goal is to learn to make room for anxiety and to continue moving toward your values even when it is present.

These are not just minor differences in technique; they are two fundamentally different ways of understanding and approaching psychological suffering.

The Importance of a Diverse Toolkit

If there is one central message to take away from this book, it is this: **there is no one right way to heal**. The human mind is incredibly complex, and the idea that a single therapeutic approach could be the perfect solution for everyone is simply not realistic. For too long, the world of therapy has sometimes been divided into competing camps, with each one arguing that its way is the best way. The future of effective therapy lies in moving beyond this rigid, one-size-fits-all mentality.

The future is about having a **diverse toolkit**. It's about recognizing that different people need different tools at different times.

- The person who is plagued by a single, deeply believed obsession might need the logical, structured tools of **I-CBT** to help them dismantle that belief and find their footing in reality again.

- The person who is struggling with a lifetime of avoiding all forms of discomfort might need the compassionate, mindfulness-based tools of **ACT** to help them open up to their experience and build a more meaningful life.

- And, as we've seen, many people might benefit from a thoughtful **integration** of both, using the tools of I-CBT to stabilize their symptoms and the tools of ACT to build long-term resilience.

An effective therapist in the 21st century is not a purist who adheres to only one model. They are a skilled craftsperson with a well-stocked toolkit, who can thoughtfully select the right tool for the right job, in collaboration with the person they are trying to help. And as someone seeking help, you are empowered when you know that you have options. If one approach doesn't feel right for you, it doesn't mean you are broken or that therapy can't help. It just means you might need a different tool.

Future Directions

The field of cognitive and behavioral therapy is constantly growing and changing. What was once a single, unified approach (CBT) has now branched out into a rich and diverse family of therapies, including I-CBT, ACT, and many others. This is an incredibly exciting time.

Here are a few of the future directions we can expect to see:

- **More Research on Personalization:** We will see more research that moves beyond the question of "Which therapy is best?" and starts to ask, "Which therapy is best for whom, and under what circumstances?" This will help us get much better at matching people with the therapeutic approach that is most likely to help them.

- **Increased Integration:** The trend toward integrating different therapeutic models will likely continue. Therapists will become more skilled at blending the wisdom of different approaches to create truly personalized treatment plans.

- **Technology and Accessibility:** The use of technology to deliver therapy, such as through internet-based programs (iCBT), will continue to grow. This will make powerful, evidence-based therapies more accessible and affordable for people all over the world. Research has already shown that iCBT can be highly effective for a range of conditions, and this is a trend that is only going to accelerate.

- **A Focus on Processes of Change:** Researchers are becoming less interested in just the brand names of therapies and more interested in the underlying *processes* that lead to change. They are asking questions like, "What are the core skills that help people get better, regardless of the therapeutic model?" This focus on common processes will help us build even more effective and efficient therapies in the future.

What all of this means for you is that there has never been a better time to seek help for your mental health. The options are more diverse, the tools are more powerful, and our understanding of the human mind is deeper than ever before. The journey out of suffering is not about finding a magic bullet, but about finding the right tools and the right guide to help you build a life of your own choosing. Whether you choose to dismantle, to defuse, or to do a little of both, the path to a freer, more flexible, and more meaningful life is open to you.

Appendices

Appendix A: Comparison Table (I-CBT vs. ACT)

Domain	Inference-Based Cognitive Behavioral Therapy (I-CBT)	Acceptance and Commitment Therapy (ACT)
Core Philosophy	Truth & Logical Validity	Workability & Values
Stance on Thoughts	A faulty conclusion to be dismantled and proven false.	A mental event to be observed and unhooked from.
Primary Goal	To resolve the obsessional doubt.	To increase psychological flexibility.
Approach to Reality	Re-establish trust in objective, sensory reality.	Accept all present-moment experience (internal & external).
Role of Anxiety	A secondary problem to be eliminated.	A normal part of life to be accepted.
Mechanism of Change	Cognitive insight (knowing before doing).	Behavioral experience (doing before knowing).
Therapist's Role	Collaborative Detective & Teacher.	Compassionate Coach & Guide.
Homework Style	Structured, skill-building worksheets and logs.	Value-driven, experiential behavioral experiments.

Appendix B: Sample I-CBT Clinician Scripts and Client Handouts

Handout: Differentiating Normal Doubts vs. Obsessional Doubts

When a doubt pops into your head, ask yourself these two questions to figure out what kind of doubt it is.

1. Is this doubt based on my senses in the here and now?

- **Normal Doubt:** Yes. It's based on real information (or a lack of it). *Example: "I can't remember if I locked the door because I was distracted by a phone call while I was leaving."*

- **Obsessional Doubt:** No. It's based on an imaginary "what if" story, even though my senses tell me everything is okay. *Example: "I saw myself lock the door, but what if the lock is broken and I didn't notice?"*

2. What happens when I check?

- **Normal Doubt:** The doubt goes away and I feel resolved. *Example: I go back and see the door is locked, and I can move on with my day.*

- **Obsessional Doubt:** The doubt might go away for a minute, but it comes right back because it was never about the door. *Example: I check the door and feel better for a moment, but then my mind says, "But what if you didn't check it well enough?"*

Clinician Script: Introducing the Obsessional Narrative

"It seems like when that doubt shows up, it's not just a single thought. It's more like a whole movie starts playing in your head. It has a plot, characters, and a lot of convincing-sounding evidence. In I-CBT, we call this the 'obsessional narrative' or the 'OCD story.' For our work together, we're not going to try to argue with this story. Instead, we're going to become experts on it. We're going to put on our detective hats and map it out, piece by piece. We want to see exactly how it's built, so we can start to see it for what it is: a very creative but ultimately fictional story."

Appendix C: Sample ACT Metaphors and Experiential Exercises

Metaphor: The Tug-of-War with a Monster

"Imagine you are in a tug-of-war with a big, ugly anxiety monster. You are pulling on the rope with all your might, and the monster is pulling back just as hard. In between you is a giant, bottomless pit. You are exhausted, and your whole life has become about this struggle. You're not going anywhere; you're just stuck in this endless fight.

What if you just... dropped the rope?

The monster would still be there, but you would no longer be in a struggle with it. You would have all of your energy back to do something else, something more important. Acceptance in ACT is like dropping the rope. It's not about defeating the monster; it's about ending the struggle so you can get on with your life."

Experiential Exercise: The "Milk, Milk, Milk" Exercise for Defusion

This exercise shows how words can lose their meaning when you change the context.

1. **Pick a negative self-judgment** that often gets you stuck (e.g., "I'm broken").

2. **Say the word out loud** for 30 seconds, but say it as quickly as you can, over and over, without pausing (e.g., "Brokenbrokenbrokenbroken...").

3. **Notice what happens.** For most people, the word starts to sound like a strange noise. The painful meaning that was attached to it starts to fall away, and you are left with just the sound. This is defusion in action. It's a demonstration that the power of a thought is not in the word itself, but in the meaning we get fused with.

Appendix D: Recommended Training Resources for I-CBT and ACT

For clinicians and individuals who wish to learn more, here are some excellent resources for further training and information.

For I-CBT:

- **The Official I-CBT Website (icbt.online):** This is the central hub for I-CBT, offering client worksheets, information on the treatment modules, and a list of trained clinicians who provide consultation and training.

- **The International OCD Foundation (IOCDF):** The IOCDF has a special interest group for I-CBT and often features webinars and conference presentations on the topic. Their website is a great source of information.

- **Clinician-Led Trainings:** Many experienced I-CBT clinicians, such as Catherine Goldhouse, offer specialized training courses for therapists. These courses often provide a deep dive into the practical application of the model.

For ACT:

- **The Association for Contextual Behavioral Science (ACBS):** This is the official organization for ACT. Their website (contextualscience.org) is a treasure trove of resources, including articles, training events, and a directory of ACT therapists around the world.

- **Books by Steven C. Hayes:** The co-founder of ACT, Steven Hayes, has written several excellent books for both clinicians and the general public. *Get Out of Your Mind and Into Your Life* is a classic self-help workbook, and *Acceptance and Commitment Therapy: The Process and Practice of Mindful Change* is the foundational text for therapists.

- **Online Training Platforms:** Many online platforms offer introductory and advanced courses in ACT for both professionals and the public.

Reference

- Aardema, F., O'Connor, K. P., & colleagues. (2022). Evaluation of Inference-Based Cognitive-Behavioral Therapy for Obsessive-Compulsive Disorder: A multicenter randomized controlled trial with three treatment modalities. *Psychotherapy and Psychosomatics, 91*(5), 348–362. https://doi.org/10.1159/000524425

- Anxiety and Depression Association of America. (2023, October 23). *Inferential confusion: A new treatment target for OCD.* https://adaa.org/learn-from-us/from-the-experts/blog-posts/consumer/inferential-confusion-new-treatment-target-ocd

- ClinicalTrials.gov. (2021). *Evaluation of a Cognitive Therapy (Inference-Based-Therapy) for the Treatment of Obsessive-Compulsive Disorder* (Identifier: NCT01794156). https://clinicaltrials.gov/study/NCT01794156

- Hayes, S. C., Strosahl, K. D., & Wilson, K. G. (2016). *Acceptance and commitment therapy: The process and practice of mindful change* (2nd ed.). The Guilford Press. (Paperback ed. 2016; hardcover first published 2011.)

- International OCD Foundation. (n.d.). *Inference-Based Cognitive-Behavioral Therapy (I-CBT)*. https://iocdf.org/ocd-treatment-guide/i-cbt/

- Julien, D., O'Connor, K. P., & Aardema, F. (2016). The inference-based approach to obsessive–compulsive disorder: A comprehensive review of its etiological model, treatment efficacy, and model of change. *Journal of Affective Disorders, 202*, 187–196

- O'Connor, K. P., Aardema, F., Bouthillier, D., Fournier, S., Guay, S., Robillard, S., Pélissier, M.-C., Landry, P., Todorov, C., Tremblay, M., & Pitre, D. (2005). Evaluation of an inference-based approach to treating obsessive-compulsive disorder. *Cognitive Behaviour Therapy, 34*(3), 148–163.

- Rozental, A., Shafran, R., Wade, T. D., Egan, S. J., Kothari, R., Ekberg, L., Wiss, M., Carlbring, P., & Andersson, G. (2017). A randomized controlled trial of Internet-Based Cognitive Behavior Therapy for perfectionism including an investigation of outcome predictors. *Behaviour Research and Therapy, 95*, 79–86.

- Shafran, R., Wade, T. D., Egan, S. J., Kothari, R., Allcott-Watson, H., Carlbring, P., Rozental, A., & Andersson, G. (2017). Is the devil in the detail? A randomised controlled trial of guided internet-based CBT for perfectionism. *Behaviour Research and Therapy, 95*, 99–106.

- Wolf, N., van Oppen, P., Hoogendoorn, A. W., van den Heuvel, O. A., van Megen, H. J. G. M., Broekhuizen, A., Kampman, M., Cath, D. C., Schruers, K. R. J., van Es, S. M., Opdam, T., van Balkom, A. J. L. M., & Visser, H. A. D. (2024). Inference-Based Cognitive Behavioral Therapy versus Cognitive Behavioral Therapy for Obsessive-Compulsive Disorder: A multisite randomized controlled non-inferiority trial. *Psychotherapy and Psychosomatics, 93*(6), 397–411.

www.ingramcontent.com/pod-product-compliance
Lightning Source LLC
Chambersburg PA
CBHW071232290326
41931CB00037B/2843